To Rick
Pump it up baby,
Malcolm

MASTERING
THE ART OF
WORKING OUT

D1383251

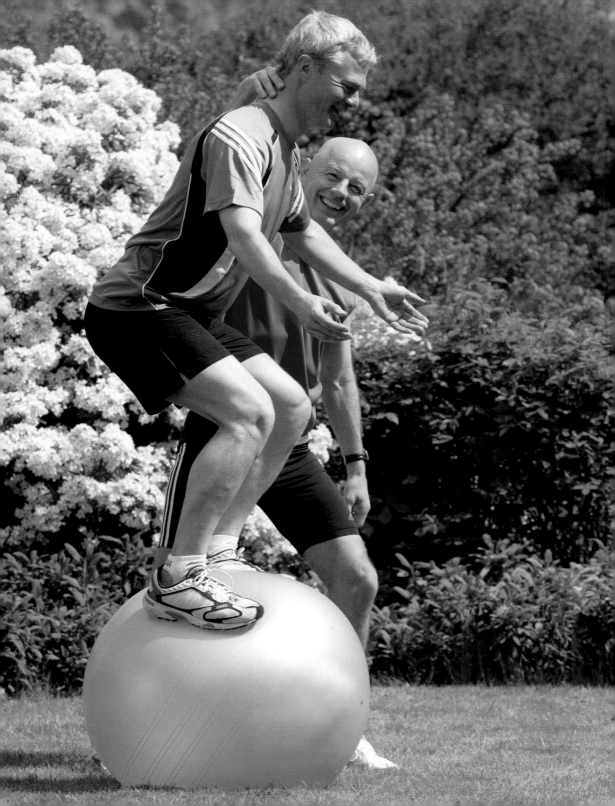

MASTERING THE ART OF WORKING OUT

Malcolm Balk and Andrew Shields

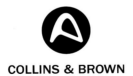

COLLINS & BROWN

First published in Great Britain in 2007 by

Collins & Brown

151 Freston Road

London

W10 6TH

An imprint of Anova Books Company Ltd

Distributed in the United States and Canada by
Sterling Publishing Co, 387 Park Avenue South,
New York, NY 10016, USA

Copyright © Collins & Brown 2007

Text copyright © Malcolm Balk and Andrew Shields 2007

The right of Malcolm Balk and Andrew Shields to be
identified as the authors of this work has been asserted
by them in accordance with the Copyright, Designs and
Patents Act 1988

All rights reserved. No part of this publication may be
reproduced, stored in a retrieval system, or transmitted in
any form or by any means, electronic, mechanical,
photocopying, recording or otherwise, without the prior
written permission of the copyright owner.

10 9 8 7 6 5 4 3 2 1

British Library Cataloguing-in-Publication Data:
A catalogue record for this book is available from the
British Library.

ISBN 1 8434 0350 1

Commissioning Editor: Victoria Alers-Hankey
Editors: Chris Stone and Fiona Corbridge
Design: Thomas Keenes
Design Manager: Gemma Wilson
Senior Production Controller: Morna McPherson
Photographs: Janie Airey

Reproduction by Anorax Printing Ltd
Printed by Craftprint International Ltd, Singapore

Acknowledgements

Thank you to everyone who has made a contribution to
this book: we really appreciate your experiences and
reflections. Thanks in particular to the following Central
YMCA staff for ongoing help and inspiration: Max Bower,
Clare Canning, Mark Harrod, Roger Mallett, David
Thompson and Brigitte Wrenn. Particular gratitude to
Robin Gargrave, director of YMCA Fitness Industry
Training, whose enthusiasm for the project was backed
up by many valuable observations on the original text.
Steven Shaw, Brita Forsstrom and Robin Simmons have
also been immensely supportive.

We would like to thank Katie Cowan and Victoria Alers-
Hankey at Anova Books for ongoing creative and
technical support; Natasha Wolek for being an excellent
'model' and Janie Airey for our fastastic photography.
This transatlantic enterprise would have been
immeasurably harder without the love and support of our
respective families: Pam and Milo, and Elaine, Helen,
Isabel and Matthew.

Malcolm Balk and Andrew Shields

CONTENTS

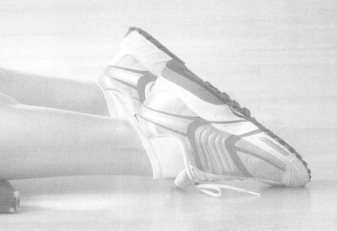

FOREWORD

By Robin Gargrave
Director, YMCA Fitness Industry Training

YMCA Fitness Industry Training has been the largest training provider for exercise and fitness instructors in the UK since its inception in 1983. The thousands of exercise instructors we have trained have been taught the principles of safe and effective exercise, a basic understanding of how the human body works, and the vital importance of teaching 'correct' technique.

However, we must ask the question: what makes an exercise 'correct'? We advocate a number of checks that an instructor can use. For example, are the muscles targeted by a resistance exercise actually doing the work without other 'helping' muscles being brought in? Are locomotory exercises free-flowing and graceful? Does an exercise take place through natural planes of movement, allowing joints and levers to follow their correct alignment?

All very good – yet we find these checks can be incredibly difficult for instructors to put into practice. Some trainee instructors have low levels of kinaesthetic awareness and may demonstrate bad habits in their own exercise technique. These habits can be tough to 'unlearn'. If we encounter such difficulties when training would-be instructors, you can imagine the problems that instructors then face when teaching their clients!

Implementing the principles of quality and effectiveness in exercise is a tremendous challenge to the fitness industry. After all, we could take the easy way out and simply ignore poor technique and inferior performance. However, the potential benefits of a more informed and thoughtful approach to exercise cannot be overestimated – which is where *Master the Art of Working Out* comes in. The aim of the book is to question the mechanical and task-oriented manner in which many people approach exercise, encouraging instead an attitude which values 'thinking in activity'. When so many people struggle to make exercise a regular part of their lives and become bored and disillusioned, this book's emphasis on gaining pleasure from the process of exercise rather than merely the end result is extremely valuable.

YMCA Fitness Industry Training is committed to getting more people more active more often, in ways that promote their health and well-being in its broadest sense. Mastering 'the art of working out' has a significant role to play in helping to achieve this.

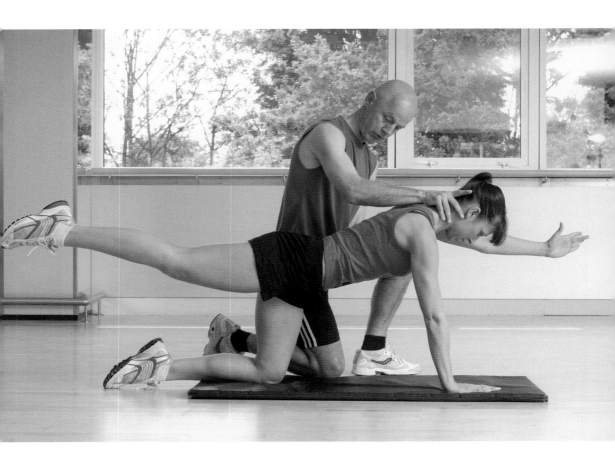

INTRODUCTION

'Fitness has to be fun. If it is not play, there will be no fitness. Play, you see, is the process. Fitness is merely the product.'

George Sheehan, cardiologist

Why do thousands of us resolve to get fit then quit our programme after a few weeks?

Why do so many people pay hundreds of pounds to join a gym then attend no more than once or twice?

Why is exercise so often described as 'boring', and considered a penance rather than a pleasure?

These are some of the questions that *Master the Art of Working Out* aims to answer.

Don't pick up this book expecting quick-fix weight-loss plans, or thoughts on the latest celebrity-endorsed routine. You know the kind of thing: 'Six weeks to a sexy new body – guaranteed!' or 'The ultimate no-sweat exercise plan'. These are part of an entirely different publishing genre – a very lucrative one, it must be said, but also one that rarely delivers results. They make fantastic promises, but demand strict adherence to rigid programmes in pursuit of difficult goals – with a yawning chasm of uncertainty between 'now' and 'then'.

The fitness world is full of such promises. Indeed, it is obsessed with measurements and targets. How often are newcomers enticed into a gym by this kind of claim: 'If you follow our routine three times a week for six months, you will lose X kg in weight, your body fat will fall by Y per cent and you will be able to wear dress size Z'? This is clever marketing talk. However, in practice it is doomed because it fails to create any engagement with the process of working out, merely setting a clutch of alluring targets somewhere in the future. It suggests that the activity is not worthwhile in itself but is merely a way to achieve something else. We exercisers are forced to pin our hopes on distant rewards without any understanding of how we're actually going to get there.

That journey, rather than the destination, is what this book is about. We see people wandering around fitness clubs with no idea what they are meant to do there. We spot others using equipment in a totally mindless, sometimes reckless, manner. And then there are those who want to get the best out of their workouts but are stuck in a comfort zone, reluctant to push themselves or to try something new and challenging. All these types of gym-goer are somewhere on the journey, but they've lost their way. This is why they are likely to give up, become bored or never reach their physical potential.

As George Sheehan noted in the quotation above, fitness has to be fun. If it is, we are more likely to stick with it and achieve results. But too few people see exercise as play – instead, they consider it work. Hard work. And, let's face it, don't we do enough of that in the rest of our lives?

Just as this is not a 'get fit quick' guide, nor is it a training manual, full of charts, schedules and those same problematic promises. Instead, it offers a new perspective on exercise and 'gym culture' through the principles of the Alexander Technique, a method of becoming aware of how we use and misuse our bodies. We will learn more about F. M. Alexander and encounter some of his ideas and procedures in the following pages – with the aim of encouraging awareness and good form whenever we lace up our trainers and begin to work out.

My story: Malcolm Balk

I first started working out in my teens, way back in the late 1960s, before gyms became the high-tech fitness centres of today. The set-up was pretty basic: free weights, benches, a few bikes and a platform to perform Olympic-type lifts. My aim was to build bigger arms, legs and chest so I could be a more intimidating ice hockey player. I was only 1.75m (5ft 9in) tall and weighed 68kg (149lb), but this did not get in the way of my quest to become a 'dominant' physical force in a sport that even then had players over 1.8m (6ft) tall, weighing at least 22kg (50lb) more than I did.

Two or three times a week I'd pump it up until, by the end of one summer, I was a massive 72kg (158lbs) with huge 34cm (13½in) arms and could bench-press nearly 89kg (200lb). When ice hockey training camp opened, I felt so strong that I went around hitting everyone, convinced I was invincible. Sadly, the dream came crashing down when I suffered a leg injury and could hardly skate, making it impossible to get close enough to unleash my devastating power. Result? I got cut from the team.

A few years later I was back in the gym, this time to improve my leg strength so I could run faster. We're now in the mid-1970s, it was the peak of the first marathon boom and I was determined to break three hours. When the first Nautilus gym opened, with its state-of-the-art machines promising unheard-of strength gains in record time, I was in there. And I must admit it was a pretty exciting place. Some of the top field-event athletes in the country trained there, huge men who could squat more than 267kg (600lb) and bench-press 222kg (500lb). Serious stuff! And here I was, a wannabe marathoner, right in the thick of it.

Although I got stronger, judging from the amount I could lift in a session, I didn't get any smarter. The cycle of injuries that had always plagued me as a runner continued. Furthermore, the tendency to go out too quickly in a marathon was exacerbated by my newfound strength. I found myself running too fast without even trying, and paying the price by the end of the race.

While all this was going on, I returned to a wholly unconnected activity from my younger days: I started playing the cello again, and several important things happened. I began to notice for the first time how much effort I put into everything I did, and realized that trying harder only made things worse.

In running and other sports, excessive tension is often masked by momentum, effort, extreme physicality and a strong urge to compete and win. However, in music, such unnecessary tension makes it almost impossible to play. It gets between you and what you want to do.

With hindsight, I now recognize that I was experiencing the same thing when it came to sport and exercise: that more was never enough, but at the same time more was too much. Thank goodness that my cello teacher at the time told me about the Alexander Technique, or I'm not sure where I would have ended up. Not only did discovering Alexander have a profound effect on the way I played the cello, it also made a dramatic difference to my running – a process described in the book *Master the Art of Running*. And, interestingly, it started to influence the way I worked out.

Before I moved to London in 1981 to begin training as an Alexander Technique teacher, my exercise schedule was a hit-or-miss affair. I worked out mainly to be better at whichever sport I was involved with at the time. So I strengthened my major muscle groups using weights, in traditional exercises such as bicep curls, dips, lat pulldowns, hamstring curls, leg extensions, squats, bench presses, and so on. I assumed that if someone had impressive arms, a massive chest or powerful-looking legs, he was obviously capable of greatness, especially when it came to competitive sport.

This assumption influenced my training, motivating me to try to develop a particular look. By copying the workouts of these supposed models of athletic wonder, I failed to find out what was really necessary to improve in my sport. I simply mimicked what was going on around me in the belief that if I did what they did, success would soon follow.

My Alexander Technique training underway, I began to question the link between particular exercises and the sport at which I was trying to improve. Would bigger hamstrings help my kick at the end of an 800m race, or larger biceps improve my second serve at tennis? More often than not, I found that the link between a particular exercise and what I wanted to develop became increasingly tenuous. Likewise, I became less preoccupied with superficial appearance. Unless you're planning a career as a lap dancer, not many people outside the locker room are going to see you naked. I realized that what Alexander Technique teachers describe as 'good use' (or what most people call 'posture') makes a far more important and long-lasting contribution to appearance (both clothed and in the buff) than pumping up your chest, tightening your butt and developing a so-called 'six-pack'.

Before I became an Alexander Technique student, the idea of 'use' meant nothing to me. I just trained hard and took pride in the effort I put into my workouts, even if a lot of it was misdirected. I still train hard, but now it's different. I take a great deal of pride in doing things that may be difficult or demanding as easily and smoothly as possible. I don't perform a set of chin-ups only with the idea of finishing it, but with the ongoing thought of how the chin-ups are affecting my use. And on those few occasions when I really go all-out and deliberately overdo it, I like to think that it's more from choice than blind habit.

We are assaulted on a daily basis, from a huge variety of sources, with information about the latest, greatest, newest and very best way to look younger instantly, run faster, lose weight, develop fab abs, and so on. The list is endless and so are the promised 'solutions'. Like many others, I too have been guilty of looking for the quick fix, the magic pill. During my three-year Alexander Technique teacher-training course, I remember

discovering the secret of teaching the Technique about once a month
during the first year. By the second year it was down to once a term. As
for the third year, it was even less often than that. Almost 20 years later, I
am still optimistic that the secret will soon be revealed! In the meantime, I
have noticed improvements in my teaching, particularly in those areas
where I've followed the principles learned many years ago. My experience
in the gym is not all that different. If I master the basics and practise them
regularly, perseverance will bring progress. Does this mean I never try
new techniques, different exercises, novel approaches? Absolutely not –
it's fun to experiment and there is always room for improvement.

Over the years, the two most important changes to my thinking about
working out are (a) that I do actually think about it and into it; and
(b) that I am more aware of the process of exercise rather than merely the
end result. Likewise, my own reasons for working out have gradually
changed. Dreams of athletic greatness have faded slightly. A 111kg
(250lb) bench press no longer holds the cachet it once did. And my self-
esteem is not as linked to the size of my biceps as it was when I was 16.
However, a workout is still an opportunity to see how well I can move,
lift, flex and coordinate myself; to push my envelope, get out of the rut
and into the groove where qualities such as connection, elasticity and skill
are valued. Even if I'm not quite as fast, strong or flexible as I used to be,
it doesn't matter.

The wonderful thing about the Alexander Technique is that not only is
it portable, it also ages well. It's still there after all these years and every
trip to the fitness centre is another chance to explore its influence in ways
that aren't part of my usual day-to-day activities.

My story: Andrew Shields

As a sport and fitness writer, I'm often asked about my own workout schedule. When I reply that I take some form of exercise most days of the week, the usual comment is: 'I suppose you have to for your job.' That's true – but it's not the reason why I'm in the gym or out on a court, pitch or track. The real explanation is simple: because I enjoy it.

'Pleasure' is an underused word when it comes to exercise. People usually mention weight loss and muscle gain, or point to their flabby bits if pressed for the reasons why they work out. As for motivation, the initial impetus often comes from a stern-talking medical practitioner or a partner concerned that they're now living with twice the person they once were. Hence the common obsession with end results and a narrow, mechanical and prescriptive approach, which can be both tedious and self-defeating.

My main enjoyment comes from the process of exercise: the challenge of learning a new routine in a dance class, of trying to bench-press a heavier weight without creating patterns of tension throughout my body, of exploring the possibilities for 'good use' while perched on a gym ball. Yes, I get a sweat up and still experience the endorphin high that comes from lifting my heart rate into the training range for half an hour or so. But my main reaction is to think: 'That was fun. I'm looking forward to doing it again soon. But first, I'll do something different tomorrow.'

'Cross-training' is the term for this kind of varied workout programme. Its aim is to alleviate boredom and reduce injury by eliminating the repetitive use of muscle groups, joints and ligaments. Why, then, when most large fitness centres offer an abundance of activities and there's also the great outdoors to explore, do so many people never veer from the routine they were given on the day they joined the club? I'm sure that if my workout schedule was an unchanging 20 minutes on the treadmill, ten minutes on the rowing machine and a prescribed route around the resistance machines, I'd have given up years ago.

It was through sport that I came upon the Alexander Technique. I heard about Steven Shaw's work linking the Technique with swimming (see p.153) and went for lessons. Although I could swim reasonable distances, my technique was poor. I envied those sleek specimens who reeled off the lengths without raising a ripple while I was a typical thrasher, wasting energy and getting nowhere.

Shaw not only altered my swimming style, he also changed my awareness of what it felt like to be in water. In practical terms, by teaching me to look at the bottom of the pool, I released the tension from my neck and shoulders. This helped to stop my body sinking and, allied to a more efficient breathing pattern, halved the number of strokes it took to complete a length. But it was his insistence that swimming should be considered an art with qualities of grace, flow, economy and sensuousness that struck me most. I'd never heard it discussed in this way.

Steven introduced me to Malcolm Balk, who was taking a similar approach to the Alexander Technique and running, and we began work on changing my mindset from that of a former sprinter and jumper – particularly a tendency to pull my head back and compress the vertebrae in my neck – to someone seeking to run for pleasure and avoid injury. The sense of ease and freedom this gave made sense when I began taking Alexander Technique lessons and continued trying to conquer what I came to learn was called 'end-gaining'. I discovered the importance of keeping my whole body flexible and poised, so I could choose how best to use it according to what I was doing.

These lessons offered a fresh insight into my sport and fitness activities. Now, when I am in the gym, I gain immense satisfaction from trying to make every lift or move perfect. And if I'm tired or pressed for time, I won't agonize about skipping a few reps and heading for the shower. I still get a kick from working out and, so long as I keep my brain switched on while I'm doing it, I hope that will never change.

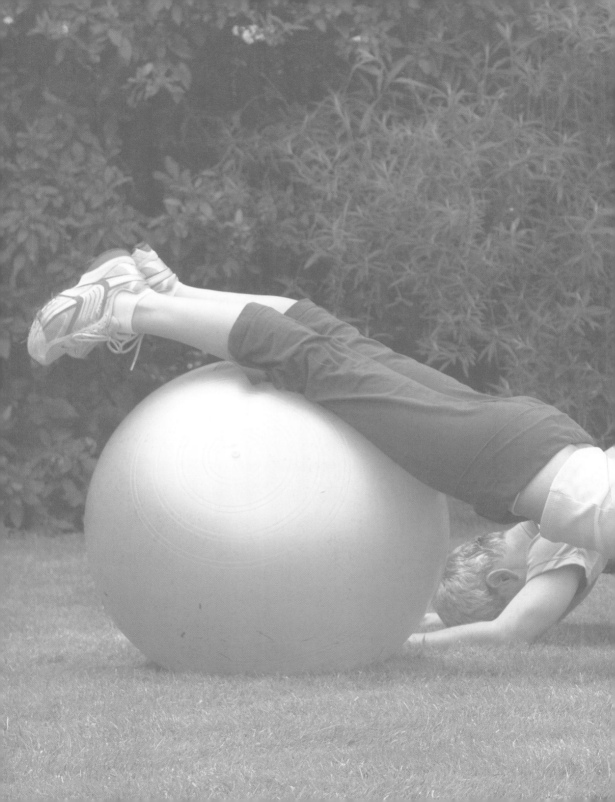

GOOD USE AND GOOD MECHANICS

'You must entice your body to cooperate. This requires patience, mindfulness and humility, three qualities often hard to access in the gym environment.'

Barefoot Doctor

1

Muhammad Ali's claim to 'float like a butterfly, sting like a bee' is more than a great quotation. It encapsulates the fact that the world's most famous boxer could not have unleashed so many telling punches without having superb balance, poise, grace, efficiency and kinaesthetic awareness. Ali was a magnificent example of an athlete possessed of something which, in the Alexander Technique, is known as 'good use'.

We can all appreciate such perfect form, whether it's displayed by a boxer, footballer, swimmer, tennis player, skater, athlete or dancer. Think of Haile Gebrselassie or any number of other African runners, Torville and Dean, Fred Astaire, Carl Lewis, Ronaldo, Ian 'Thorpedo' Thorpe, Margot Fonteyn or Roger Federer: these sportspeople and performers make the impossible look easy.

It's common to hear exercise professionals and sports coaches describe athletes as having 'good mechanics'. By this they usually mean someone who demonstrates a high level of skill, has excellent technique and who moves smoothly and efficiently. This is a subject which can get seriously complicated: read just a little about how biomechanists describe technique and you're into kinematics and kinetics, appropriate forces being applied in the right direction, muscles firing in the correct combinations and sequences, and so on.

We are right to pay such close attention to form, so let's keep it simple. After all, it's fair to assume that most of us don't just want to get in shape but to continue doing so in a sustainable way once the original euphoria has worn off. Furthermore, we know that exercising in an uncoordinated and inefficient manner increases the risk of injury.

At the heart of the Alexander Technique is a belief that 'use' affects functioning. In other words, it's vital to consider how we do things, not just what we do. For some people, merely shifting their butt into the gym is a major accomplishment, while actually joining a class or lifting a few weights may be cause for major celebration. However, for the greater number who exercise regularly but find their fitness levels reaching a plateau and notice an increase in persistent niggles, the issue is more serious. This is why it's important to pay attention to use.

A large part of any fitness professional's training is spent learning how to perform given exercises correctly, then how to convey that information to the public. However, much of this knowledge is wasted, misinterpreted and ignored. Why is this?

Given the size of popular group exercise classes, which often have more than 30 participants, there is little or no time for individual feedback. People are mostly

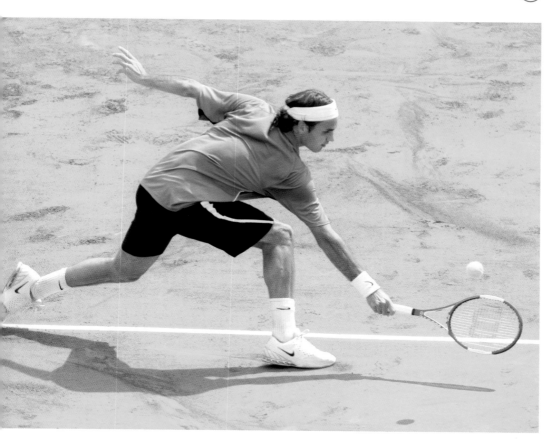

left to their own devices. For a proportion of those taking part, simply doing the class is enough – they aren't concerned with form (often until it's too late). In contrast, the majority do try to follow the instructions and example provided by the teacher. Yet the difference between the movements/instructions of the teacher and what happens among the participants can be enormous. Assuming that everyone is trying their best to follow the leader, this is cause for some concern. What we think or feel is happening may be quite different from the reality. You may believe you're 'Ms Step Aerobics 2007' but a glance in the mirror or a peek at yourself on video often tells a completely different tale.

When an instructor encourages class members to 'Keep your back straight' and perhaps provides an example, most people assume not only that they can do it, but that their idea of straight is straight. This isn't always so: ask a friend to

Above Tennis great Roger Federer, whose grace, efficiency and kinaesthetic awareness make the impossible look easy.

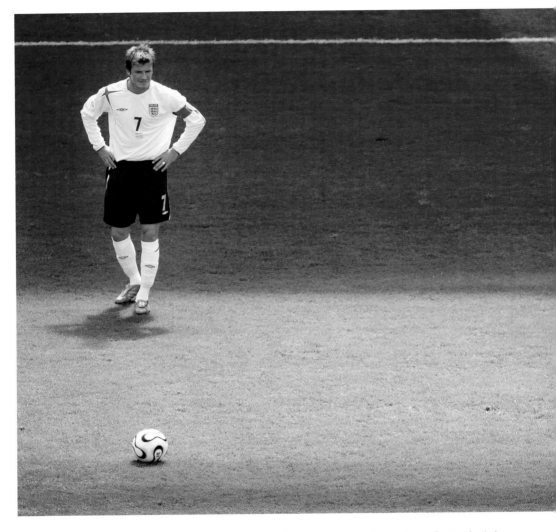

stand straight (that is, vertically) and nine times out of ten you'll find he tends to lean backwards. He'll also be prepared to swear that when he stands against a wall, he is leaning forwards. So how does a teacher with 30 eager exercisers correct this situation? Often with well-intentioned, yet potentially harmful advice like: 'Pull in your belly button', 'Tighten your buttocks', 'Pull your shoulders back' or 'Tuck in your chin.' It's the classic 'outside-in' approach loved by army drill sergeant majors the world over: freedom sacrificed for the sake of form.

Above Former England football captain David Beckham shows the importance of balance, poise and lots of 'up' in preparation for the precision skill of taking a free kick.

Talent, technique and use

'Talent' is what we're born with. It's our potential. 'Technique' is the know-how needed to perform a movement or activity. 'Use' is the way we do things, with specific awareness of the relationship between our head, neck and back. The three concepts are not synonymous.

Some people with God-given talent can fall out of bed with a stinking hangover and still dunk a basketball or do the splits as if it's no big deal. Many sportspeople and fitness instructors who don't have particularly good use have developed high levels of skill in their particular activity. For example, footballers may hunch their backs and tighten their shoulders but, despite 'misusing' themselves in these ways, they can still control a ball with great skill and precision. In contrast, a person can have good use but lack the technique or skill needed to perform a power clean or get to grips with a complicated dance routine.

Is there a link between good use and good form? Sometimes, but not always. Take the example of alignment. We are often urged to think about showing 'proper alignment' when we exercise. This usually means stacking things up on top of each other so we are in better balance. However, the example of the drill sergeant major shows that what is conventionally thought of as 'proper alignment' can only be achieved at considerable expense.

Use implies freedom, and freedom is a condition, not a position. In the gym, some people look slim, trim and well muscled, but their bodies betray great rigidity: their joints are stiff so whatever they do requires more effort than the results warrant. This is an example of good alignment with poor use.

So where does this leave us? Talent is something we all have to some degree. We don't have any say in the amount of talent we're blessed with, but bad use will undoubtedly limit our ability to develop it fully. However, technical skill can be learned and good use can be worked on and improved. They are both within our sphere of influence.

If you don't have the genetic make-up to be a world-class athlete, dancer or gymnast, no amount of good use will make you one. It's the same in the gym: some people are born to hoist very heavy weights above their head with ease, others to place their head on their knee with relative ease. For we lesser mortals, the Alexander Technique and its principle of good use will enhance any activity to which it is applied. It makes it easier to assimilate new skills and helps us develop our potential. And it makes the whole business of learning a lot less painful and much more fun.

Learning new skills

What most of us do when we try to learn a new routine in an exercise to music class, or develop appropriate technique on a resistance machine, is to focus on the parts of the body most involved in the activity: thus, in the case of a step workout, the feet. Unfortunately, this is a short-sighted method as it can cause us to miss seeing the forest for the trees. Merely focusing on specific body parts may lead to, say, the leg making a better movement – but unless this thinking is connected to the whole, there will be a lack of context and overall meaning. It's like learning to pronounce the words of a foreign language without knowing their meaning.

Here are two scenarios from a step class in which individuals with equal talent try it for the first time:

Dave is a real goer who decides that a step class is just the ticket to losing that extra weight he put on over the holidays. He's

Below The instability of a gym ball poses a challenge to our ability to maintain length in activity.

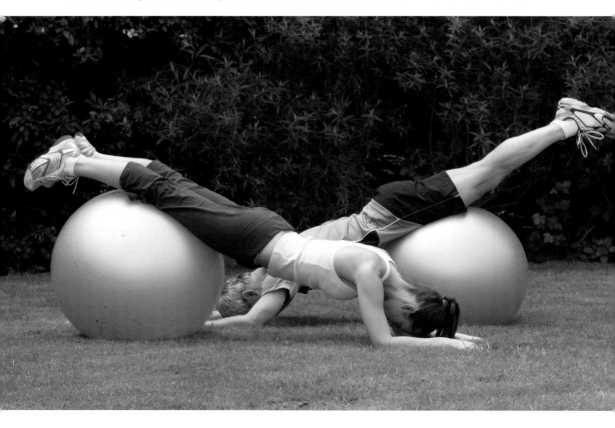

a gym regular, has always believed in working hard and reckons he'll sort this class out in short order. When some of the steps seem trickier than expected he's a little surprised but pushes on, certain that things will improve. However, he always seems to be behind everyone else. Instead of moving smoothly and rhythmically, he's a bit of a heavy stepper.

Figuring that the secret is in the footwork, Dave tries in vain to master the intricate steps of the instructor. But whenever he focuses on the foot movements, he loses the beat. His body doesn't seem to be very well coordinated. He leans too far back and tends to strain, particularly in the shoulder area. This results in the back of his neck shortening, which makes him resemble a turtle. He leaves the class tired and frustrated at his lack of progress.

Dan is a new member at the gym and tries the step class in a spirit of adventure. He has never been much of a mover and, within a few minutes, realizes the sequences are too difficult for him. He makes a key decision: he'll stop trying to keep up but he won't quit, and decides instead to learn one thing well. He'll master a basic step-up and step-down pattern, to the rhythm; the turns and side-steps can be left for the moment.

Dan practises a few steps in the mirror on his own. He soon notices that if his foot leads the step-up, he leans backwards and his neck tightens, creating strain there and into his shoulders. He also reasons that it is better to lead with the knee rather the foot when walking or climbing stairs. Trying this brings better results. His neck no longer tightens and he steps up more smoothly, especially when the lower foot helps at the last moment with a little push from the toes. As for stepping down, he finds he can lessen the impact if he 'thinks up' as his foot touches the ground. This seems to prevent all his weight from crashing on to the landing foot and helps to develop a greater sense of flow and lightness.

Experimenting with the movement of his arms, Dan finds he can control the rhythm of his feet indirectly: speed up the arms and the feet seem to follow. This makes it easier for him to stay with the beat. All the time he makes sure that his head remains poised, neither flopping around nor held rigidly in place. Whenever things get difficult he returns to establishing a balanced head-neck-back relationship and it seems easier to get on track again.

Once the mechanics of the basic step have been mastered, Dan sets himself a realistic goal: he'll learn one tricky move per class. The rest of the time he'll just keep up with the basic step, which still gives him a good workout but allows a chance to focus on what the instructor is doing. At the end of each class he asks for and receives a little feedback on the development of his newest step, and he takes a few minutes during the next week to practise slowly so that he grooves it before moving on.

Will it be Dave or Dan who sticks with the step class and gains increasing pleasure – not to mention fitness – from taking part? The answer is obvious. Learning to marry good use to good mechanics is the ideal way to develop skill and maintain interest.

The 'new gym'

Over the last decade, restaurant diners on both sides of the Atlantic have grown accustomed to the concept of 'fusion food'. Ingredients, ideas and inspiration are drawn from every part of the globe to create dishes that excite the imagination as well as the palate. Critics claim that an approach which mixes a little bit of this and a little bit of that can lack rigour and depth of knowledge, but enthusiasts insist it's a sign of gastronomic maturity that we're willing to be so bold and experimental in what we eat.

Over the same period, the exercise industry has begun a similar process of exploration into what might be termed 'fusion fitness'. This is based on a recognition that training methods from very different cultures have similar objectives. At the heart of both ancient Eastern and more contemporary Western techniques are a desire for efficient, effective and aesthetically pleasing movement, and the cultivation of muscular strength and endurance, flexibility, coordination, balance and 'internal energy'. Together, these support the belief that true fitness requires workouts for the body, the mind and the spirit.

In an attempt to develop this more holistic approach to fitness, most gym timetables now feature yoga, tai chi, Pilates and various martial arts. Instead of an unrelenting diet of cardiovascular machines, circuit training, spinning and weights, exercisers are being encouraged into a programme that presents a wider range of physical and mental challenges. It's evident from the clamour for classes that this is far more than just the latest fad.

With its 2,000-year history, myriad styles, spiritual underpinning and celebrity endorsement from the likes of Sting and Christy Turlington, yoga was always going to appeal to jaded gym-goers. Meanwhile, the equally ancient, gentle, graceful and meditative movements of tai chi provide a way for us to relax and rebalance our *chi* (vitality). Of more recent techniques, Pilates has moved from being a system known only to ballet dancers and athletes to a hugely popular method of satisfying the current obsession with core stability, using exercises that are, in effect, training from the inside outward. Finally, martial arts offer the complete package of oriental philosophy, body-mind awareness, self-defence, meditation, breathing techniques and a tough cardiovascular workout with the option of physical contact.

A recognition that, for example, yoga and weight training are mutually beneficial is described by world-renowned yoga teacher Baron Baptiste in his book, *Journey into Power*: 'On a recent trip to Los Angeles, I went to one of my old haunts, Gold's Gym, in Venice Beach. That particular gym is like the world mecca of bodybuilding. Arnold [Schwarzenegger] trained there, as have countless others. When I told a friend where I'd gone, she laughed and said: "I love it. The big yogi pumps iron?" "It's all yoga," I told her. "On or off the mat, it's yoga."

'Even if I'm in the crème de la crème of the weightlifting world, I'm still putting all I have learned in my practice into action. I'm using my *ujjayi* breathing for stamina and presence, my abdominal lock for core stabilization, a focused gaze for calm determination, the Master Principles of Alignment for healthy form. Yes, I'm lifting weights, but beyond that I stay aware of my edge, practise maintaining equanimity, and use my intuition to know when less is more and when to push further.'

In some fitness clubs you will find classes devoted to a 'pure' form of these pursuits. As an alternative, you might come across 'Yogilates', 'Body Combat', 'Cardio Kick', 'Thai-Bo' or other branded workouts which draw on the principles outlined above but are moulded into marketable packages. These often give an excellent introduction to the various disciplines, but should never be taken for 'the real thing'. What's more, the relatively small amount of training needed to teach such workouts can irritate instructors who have undergone long courses of study in their specialist discipline. Even so, it's undeniable that 'the new gym' gives exercisers greater variety and stimulation than ever before – and a far wider range of reasons to persevere with a fitness programme.

Though yoga, tai chi, Pilates and martial arts are talked of as 'body-mind' techniques, this is no guarantee that they will be performed in anything other than the same mechanical and mindless fashion found elsewhere in the gym. What we are seeking instead is the intelligent approach that can be developed through an appreciation of the Alexander principles. Throughout this book you will find case studies in which specialist instructors and exercisers address this issue.

Yoga

*'I listen to the instructions given by the teacher.
Then I ask myself: what do I actually need to do?'*

When I began taking yoga classes, five mornings a week, I always placed myself in the front row in order to catch the teacher's energy. I reminded myself that at any time I could modify my activity level. I decided to disregard those students in the rows behind; however, they were 'there' and I secretly wanted to be 'good'. I thought that because I had been a dancer this would be easy.

Each time the teacher led us into an asana – into a convoluted, distorted, backwards, twisted, upside-down posture – I felt sure I would break! Finally, I told myself that people had been doing yoga for thousands of years and they hadn't broken. But this was pain, which caused my mind to be in a thousand places at once and I had no idea where my body was in space. In order to 'do it right', I cultivated muscular effort.

I struggled to do what I was told. I would hear only a stream of instructions: 'Pull your wing bones back and down, root your feet into the floor, lift the quadriceps and resist with the calf muscle to keep the knees from hyper-extending, rotate the right waist forward and the left waist toward the back of the room to bring the trunk in line with the median plane of the body. Move the back spine in and up to open the frontal chest as you move the shoulders down. Breathe through your legs!' When I was standing in a posture, the teacher would adjust my already tightened predicament, adding another layer of effort. I didn't even notice that sometimes the teacher gave incorrect anatomical references.

At first it seemed inconceivable that I could think of yoga as an activity, like I did with walking or sitting when I was in my Alexander

Technique class. It was just so hard to think at all and do what I wanted to. How could I reconcile the language of yoga with the language – the sequence of thinking – of the Alexander Technique? Because yoga is such a venerated institution, who was I to dare to criticize it in any way?

I demonstrated asanas in my Alexander Technique class. My teacher and classmates helped me reorder my thinking. I learned to pay attention to my whole self first, to the relationship of my head to my body, in order to avoid extra tightening that interfered with my natural coordination. I found that I could move more easily, further. What's more, it was fun! However, it was difficult to apply this new sequence of thinking about how to move efficiently when I was being given other instructions during a yoga class.

Gradually, I have managed to pay attention to my thinking whenever it occurs to me. I listen to the instructions given by the teacher. Then I ask myself: what do I actually need to do? If it's a twist, I can choose to lead with my head first, even if instructed to 'rotate the chest'. I think of the words as if they were people on a crowded street; I am aware of them but I can choose to let them pass. If, in the middle of an asana, I notice that I have skipped ahead or I am in pain, I simply ask again, always considering the relationship of my head to my body first. No one ever seems to mind.

One day, I made a huge discovery. The language of yoga only refers to parts. Alexander Technique considers the whole body in movement. As I remember this difference while I am in class, it makes it much easier for me to reinterpret the language of the yoga instruction for myself. I know that I'm safer if I take a split second to attend to this re-evaluation. I am not rebelling at yoga: I'm being smart about my own self by not working harder than I need to.

Carol Levin

A teacher's experience

'He had been using a tight body badly.'

For many people who practise the Alexander Technique, sport and fitness activities play an important role in their lives. In exercising, we feel satisfied that we are doing something towards maintaining our health and preventing disease. Working out can also be good fun.

Some pupils initially have very little awareness that the Technique can help them perform better in the gym and reduce the risk of injury. They may have booked a lesson because they have heard that it will help them with, for example, their back and postural problems. Soon, however, they start to recognize that these problems have their origins in how they are misusing themselves in all daily activity. From there develops an understanding that this misuse is taken with them into the gym, where it becomes intensified and exaggerated.

In an ideal world, we would start applying the Technique to our physical activities before any problems manifested themselves. After all, prevention is always better than cure. Unfortunately, as in the case of Mike, it's not until our attention is drawn to the alerting messages of pain that we consider changing the way we go about things.

Mike had been forced to take early retirement from his career as a bank manager because of chronic back pain. An intelligent man in his late 50s, he was committed to helping himself recover. He had been seeing a physiotherapist for 18 months prior to his first Alexander Technique lesson and had been carrying out the various recommended exercises, but was frustrated because he was still very limited in what he could do. Wanting to maintain a fulfilling and active retirement (he is a keen gardener), Mike's best strategy had been to do as much as he could, when he could, knowing there would be a price to pay.

During his first lesson, the muscular release achieved in Mike's back enabled a different way of breathing, which was much freer than anything he had experienced for some time. At this point, he noted that one of the strategies he had used for coping with the pain had been to tighten and 'fix' in his whole body. A consequence of this was much shallower breathing. Encouraged by this improvement, Mike enthusiastically started applying what he was learning in his Alexander lessons and began to change his approach to gardening. He would take more time to think about what he was going to do and break down each task into smaller, more manageable units, working continuously with more consciousness about how he was using himself.

It wasn't until one day during a lesson, when I asked him to release his ankles, that another penny dropped for Mike. He began to consider his footballing days as a younger man. He recalled that he always had tight ankles, which had caused him difficulties on the pitch. From there he began to think about his experiences in the gym: he had worked out regularly during his youth. With hindsight and the benefit of Alexander Technique lessons Mike could see that, during his gym days, he had been using a tight body badly and had placed considerable stress on his back. The gyms of 30 or 40 years ago were far cruder than today, but the ethos was the same: driving yourself harder and faster to achieve more, with little concern for the quality of a movement and the potential long-term damage that results from such misuse.

Mike appreciates that had he then possessed and applied the knowledge of how to use himself that he has today, his back problems would probably never have arisen. He recognizes that the same mindfulness which he now applies to gardening and other physical activities is especially necessary when using oneself under more extreme conditions, such as working out – or, as with his most recent project, laying a patio in his back garden. His story is a reminder of how the consequences of poor use can reveal themselves in the years to come.

Madelene Webb

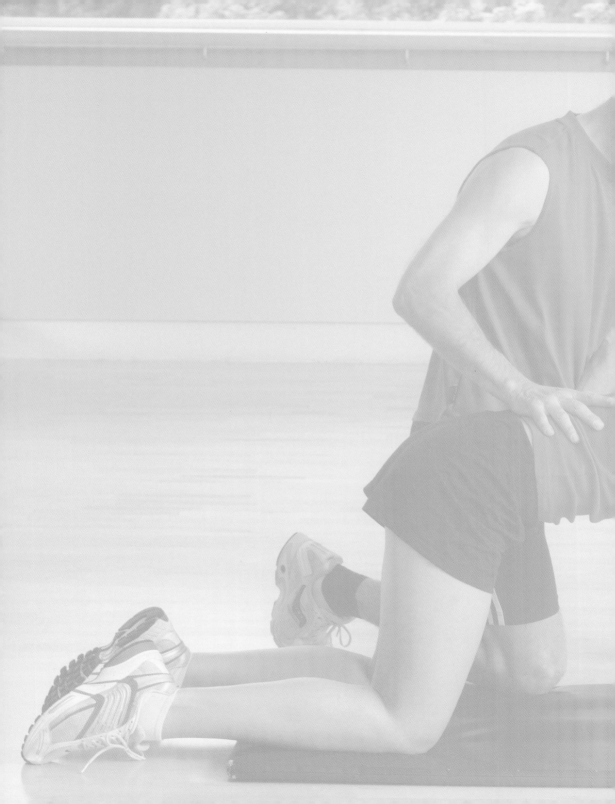

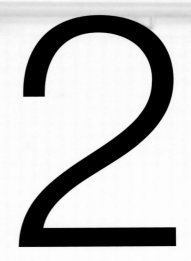

2

THOUGHTFUL
ACTIVITY

'Training was not only a matter of tensing my muscles but,
equally importantly, of relaxing them. I was not only building a
body, but also dreams.'

Sven Lindqvist, *Bench Press*

When Dave and Dan tackled their step class in Chapter 1, it was the latter who got to grips with the basic mechanics and movements by thinking through his approach. In fact, Dan was applying principles of the Alexander Technique to his workout. Who, then, was Alexander, and why are the principles he developed so useful in the gyms and fitness clubs of today?

Australia is among the world's most sporty and health-loving nations, from its all-conquering cricket and rugby teams to the swimmers and surfers who relish the superb climate and outdoor lifestyle. It has produced legendary athletes like Herb Elliott, Ron Clarke and Cathy Freeman, while generations of its top exercise professionals and sports scientists have propelled the fitness industry forward.

However, those involved in all this activity may be less familiar with another Australian, from northern Tasmania. They may wonder how an actor whose early career was plagued by chronic hoarseness and laryngitis could influence the philosophy of leading fitness experts and sports coaches.

Frederick Matthias Alexander (1869–1955) specialized in dramatic and humorous monologues. His story reflects a feeling that many gym-goers, runners or games players may have had at one time or another: 'I know I can do better, so why isn't it happening for me? I have all this potential but I don't know how to realize it.' Alexander loved to perform and recite, but he suffered from a problem that prevented him doing so to the best of his ability. On stage, he would go hoarse and have to cut short his performance.

Unlike his material, this was no laughing matter. So Alexander did what most of us would have done under the circumstances: he sought advice from the medical profession, none of which was very helpful, except for the suggestion that he should rest. However, as soon as he put his voice to the test again, the hoarseness would recur.

Finally, he decided to tackle the problem himself. He reasoned that there must be a link between the way he recited and the difficulty with his voice. To find out what was happening, he set up mirrors so he could observe himself while speaking. He immediately noticed several habits that seemed worth investigating: there was an increased tension in his throat, his breathing and his neck as he began to recite. Further observation showed that these changes occurred not just when he spoke, but from the moment he started to think about speaking. 'I saw that as soon as I started to recite, I tended to pull back the head, depress the larynx and suck in breath through the mouth in such a way as to produce a gasping sound,' he later wrote. He realized that his problem was not merely physical, but involved his physical, mental and emotional make-up. In other words, his entire being was implicated.

Alexander began to explore different ways to release these tensions. Through experiments, he discovered that there was a strong interconnection between his head, neck and back – which he called 'the primary control of use'. Any interference with this relationship seemed to have an indirect effect not only on his voice but on his overall functioning. He also recognized that there was an important link between what, and how, he was thinking, and what he found himself actually doing. If he tried to correct what he observed in the mirror, for example by putting his head in a 'better position', the results were short-lived. In order to make a reliable and long-lasting change, he realized that first and foremost he had to prevent the wrong response from occurring. Mastering this skill enabled Alexander to perform without injury as well as to enjoy an improvement in his overall health.

Upon returning to the stage, he encountered other actors with similar problems to his own. He offered them advice and hands-on help, and they would improve as well. He moved to London in 1904 and developed his technique as a way of becoming aware of, and preventing, the unnecessary tension we put into everything we do, in order to function in a more free and natural fashion. Henry Irving, Lillie Langtry and Herbert Beerbohm Tree were among the many actors who later studied what became known as the Alexander Technique. Alexander continued to take on pupils – he never called them patients – including Aldous Huxley, Adrian Boult and George Bernard Shaw, the last of that trio starting lessons when he was aged 80.

John Cleese, Daley Thompson, Linford Christie and John McEnroe are more recent students of the Technique, while the Technique is also part of the curriculum at institutions ranging from the Royal Academy of the Dramatic Arts (RADA) to the American Conservatory Theater, San Francisco.

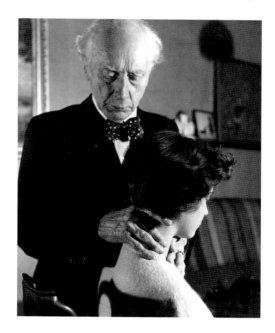

Above F. M. Alexander (1869–1955) working with a pupil to direct her head 'forward and up".

Alexander's discoveries

Alexander was neither an athlete nor a fitness buff. However, he could, in today's terms, be described as a master personal trainer. He was concerned with the 'use of the self' – a concept that emphasizes as its core message, more than any other method around then or since, the primary significance of unity of mind and body in every act we perform. To quote Sir Charles Sherrington, the winner of the 1932 Nobel Prize in physiology and medicine: 'Each waking day is a stage dominated for good or ill, in comedy, farce or tragedy, by a dramatis persona – the self. And so it will be until the final curtain drops. The self is a unity.' This has universal applications for our health and well-

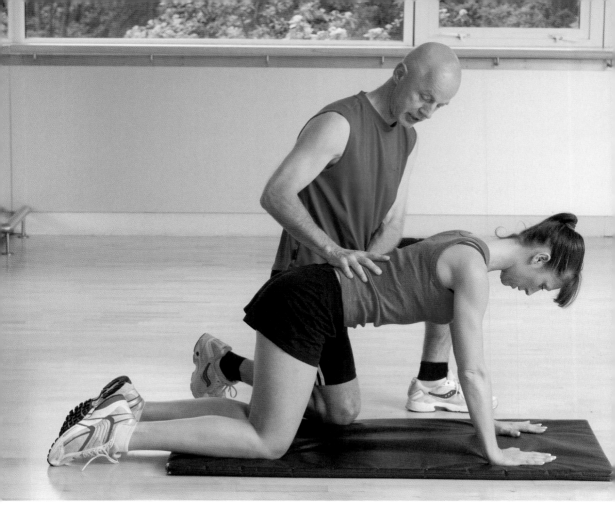

being. However, Alexander did not start out with such grandiose ambitions but, as we have seen, simply wanted to find a way to project his voice on stage without going hoarse.

From our perspective, Alexander's realization of use is extremely valuable for anyone trying to improve or maintain their fitness. 'Being in shape' is about more than how much you weigh, how long you can survive on the Stairmaster, the size of your biceps or the poundage on your bench-press bar. The way you 'use yourself' determines the

Above Here, the aim is to maintain a sense of widening in the lower back in preparation for a core stability exercise.

way you function. For example, if you regularly visit the gym and exercise to improve your posture, but spend the rest of the day slumped in front of a computer and television, which of those actions is going to have greater effect? And, to take the point even further, how much improvement can you expect to make if your slumping habit permeates every exercise you perform to 'correct' it?

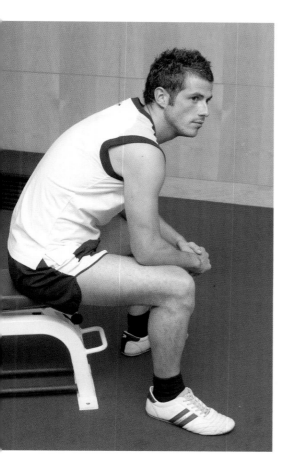

Above Recovery in between weight-training sets doesn't have to mean collapsing the body into an unthinking slump – although this is more often the rule than the exception in the gym.

The many hours Alexander spent observing himself in his quest to change the well-entrenched psychophysical pattern that threatened to end his acting career proved beyond a doubt that trying to overpower a bad habit by immediate and direct means doesn't work. What we resist persists! In other words, if you use yourself poorly while you exercise, you run the grave risk of reinforcing what you are already doing badly: practice, after all, makes permanent. To change functioning, you first need to change use, and not the other way round.

Let's employ a mechanical metaphor to make the point clear. In this life, you are both car and driver. In spite of advances in replacement technology (such as new hips and complex knee reconstructions), the original parts generally work best. So if you wreck the engine, strip the tyres, fry the brakes and stain the upholstery, you can't trade it in for a new model. As driving instructors everywhere will tell you, we all bring attitudes, skills and habits to bear on the way our car performs on the road. We pop the clutch, slam on the brakes, over-rev the engine, reverse into the kerb and fail to look in the mirror before changing lanes. All these factors contribute to the functioning of the vehicle and, ultimately, the quality of the ride.

The primary control of use

Alexander found that his vocal difficulties were related to a general pattern of interference with the natural relationship between his head, neck and back. He realized that this was the key area to focus on when 'unlearning' habitual reactions and tensions. This area exerts a powerful influence on the way we function (including, of course, the way we walk, run, lift, stand and sit). Ideally, the neck should be free of unnecessary tension – that is, not pulling the head down into the spine. The head should be poised freely on top of the spine in such a way that the spine is encouraged to lengthen and the back is encouraged to widen. This produces ease, effortlessness and a sense of lightness in movement.

Alexander was particularly concerned with the role that the neck plays in our use. More specifically, with the fact that most people over-tighten this area. It's a habit that is often overlooked by people when they work out and it can strongly influence the amount of effort exerted during any activity.

Professor Emeritus E. J. Abrahams of Queen's University in Canada, a leading medical researcher on neck muscles and their importance, insists: 'The evidence that the neck plays a critical role in posture is overwhelming.' In an experiment designed to demonstrate this fact, a volunteer had a local anaesthetic injected into one side of his neck. The loss of muscle sensation and of muscle tone on the injected side gave him the illusion of falling over to that side. The subject reported that he felt drawn to one side like an iron bar to a magnet. He was unable to walk with any coordination, like someone who has had too much alcohol. When lying down, he felt the couch was toppling over towards the side of the injection. As the late David Garlick, professor of anatomy at the University of New South Wales in Australia, pointed out in his book *The Lost Sixth Sense*: 'The dominating nerve inputs from the neck help to determine how the brain controls muscles in posture and movement.'

Another key element in Alexander's concept of good use is what he called 'quickening the mind'. It is a state of receptivity in which we are simultaneously aware of both what we are doing and how we are doing it. For example, a good driver will notice what is not happening (tailgating, speeding, leaving the indicator on, rubbernecking and so on) as well as what is (foot on the accelerator, hands on the steering wheel, proximity of other cars).

People from less industrialized nations seem not to disturb their natural use as much as we do in the West. For example, physiologists have found that Kenyan women use no more effort – that is, oxygen consumption – walking up a hill with a 10kg (22lb) jug of water balanced on their head than you or I without one. Various explanations have been proposed, but one valid theory is that Kenyan women already possess excellent balance and coordination.

Faulty sensory awareness

One of the most interesting discoveries Alexander made was that all of us tend to have a limited awareness of what we are doing. No matter the activity we are engaged in, far more is going on than we think or feel we are doing. We may habitually sit chatting to friends with our legs crossed and simply not notice that our lower back has collapsed and our breathing has been compromised. We may pick up a drink and not observe that we jut our chin forwards and sharply retract our head as our lips reach the glass – a habit that can, over

Right The aim here is to lengthen the spine and keep the hips back while performing a lunge, expanding our awareness both of what we are doing and the way we are doing it.

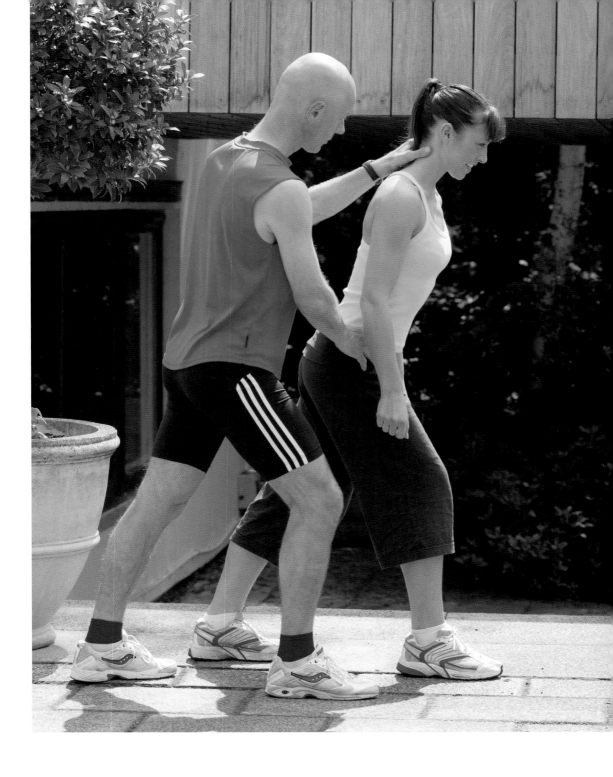

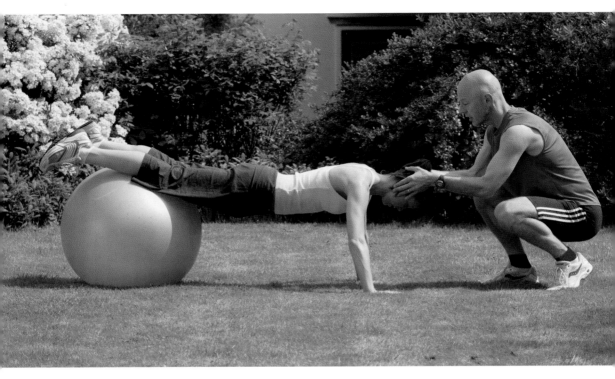

Above The head should lead the spine, which helps to maintain integrity through the core – even in this horizontal position on a gym ball.

time, create a humped back. We are not aware of these 'extra' things we are doing when we are interested in other matters like talking or drinking. It is even possible to try hard to stand up straight and tall but actually be more hollow-backed (that is, not straight) and shorter (by stiffening) than our real height – the opposite of what we feel we are doing. One of the most important factors in changing our way of doing anything is to eliminate these extra actions, which are wasteful of our energy and power.

People who see themselves on video or in photographs are often surprised at what they really look like as opposed to what they thought they looked like. It's the same when we hear our voice on an answering machine: it doesn't sound like us. This understanding is important when we try to change an ingrained habit. The new and 'improved' version often feels odd, awkward or even wrong – which increases the likelihood of going back to what we know because it feels right, even if the old way isn't serving us well.

Most of us believe that if we are told what to do – or, better still, shown – then we should be able to carry out the instructions or follow the demonstration without any trouble. Sadly, and often painfully, reality does not support this assumption. Try this simple test:

Cross your arms. Have a look at them, see which one is over and which under. Now cross them the other way. Take your time! How does the new way feel? As natural and comfortable as the first? Probably not. How likely would you be to cross your arms this way if it was the 'correct' way to perform this movement?

What can we blame for this sad state of affairs? Let's put it down to 'faulty sensory awareness'. We generally talk about having five senses – sight, smell, hearing, taste and touch. The 19th-century anatomist Charles Bell identified a sixth sense, which is commonly referred to as 'kinaesthesia' or 'proprioception'. It refers to our ability to know where one bit of our body is in relation to another, either at rest or in movement.

Faulty sensory awareness refers to the fact that when we try to correct or improve ourselves either in action or at rest, our internal guidance system – the kinaesthetic sense – cannot be relied on to provide accurate feedback. Here's a hypothetical example: you've been doing a favourite exercise to music class on a regular basis and feel you've perfected all the routines. But then the teacher tells you that your head is moving around all over the place during certain moves and you might want to think about keeping it more centred and under control. After getting over your initial shock at the comment, you do a little extra practice at home – just to fine-tune what must obviously be your instructor's compulsive pickiness for minor details. Returning triumphantly to the class, you demonstrate your newfound prowess only to be told quietly

afterwards that the head thing seems a little worse than before. You can't believe it! But when your teacher takes the time to show you in the mirror, you are mortified to realize she is right. How could this happen if you couldn't even feel it?

Alexander offered a clue when he remarked that: 'You can't know a thing by an instrument that is wrong.' The instrument to which he was referring is, of course, our kinaesthetic sense. The difficulty Alexander encountered, and which is widespread in today's society, is that the familiar becomes the standard by which we judge what is right and what is wrong. Since the exerciser in our scenario was trying hard to improve, we can guess with some certainty that she was doing what felt right – which was moving her head. The challenge, when trying to change an old habit, is to become comfortable with the unfamiliar. This is hard to do under the best of circumstances, but is particularly difficult when one is striving to 'get it right'.

Chronic tension also plays a role in faulty sensory awareness. Muscles which are tightened for long periods of time no longer provide the brain with feedback. In other words, we become less aware of what is going on in these areas, and it therefore becomes harder to make the decisions necessary to maintain our poise, balance and enjoyment – that is, to release unnecessary tension.

Recognizing habits

Whether in the weights room or dance studio, our workouts tend to follow a familiar routine. If it's the former you prefer, your schedule might look something like this: ten minutes on the bike or treadmill to warm up, then two or three sets of reps on the machines or free weights. You might end with another cycle or run, then stretch out before heading off to the shower, job done. Most exercise to music classes also use a broadly predictable structure: warm-up followed by the hard, cardio bit then a cool-down and stretch to finish.

Following a routine is not bad. Many of these sequences are based on sound physiological principles and should be respected. For the average person, the challenge of continually coming up with new routines is better left to the exercise professionals. The question, then, is how to prevent the familiar from becoming mechanical, where the predictability of a routine dulls the brain and you are no longer aware of what you're doing.

This lack of connection with what is happening in the moment has many consequences. The obvious one is boredom. However, an interesting case was cited by a doctor studying this issue. He worked with a woman who, while using an exercise bike, would become so engrossed in a book that 30 minutes would seem like only five. The problem here was that she only seemed to get five minutes' worth of benefit, no doubt because her focus was on the book and not on the effort she was expending – or, more

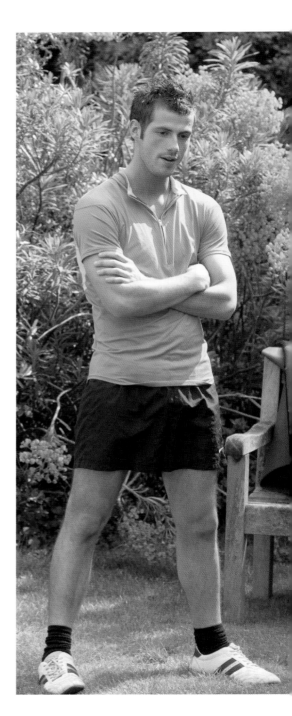

Right 'Wherever you go, there you are.' Note the knees locked, hips pushed forward, back arched, arms crossed and shoulders pulled forward and down. Is this how *you* stand when you're not 'thinking'?

probably, not expending – on the bike. After several months, her level of fitness had shown little improvement. His solution was to get her to put the book down and simply cycle, so that 30 minutes' effort actually felt like 30 minutes. When this happened, she began to make positive gains.

A study of runners carried out in the early 1990s looked at the advantages and disadvantages of running when 'associated' (switched on) and 'disassociated' (switched off). People who disassociate tend to distract themselves from discomfort, pain or tedium by thinking of something more pleasant. But runners who associate, the research showed, pay more attention to the signals coming from their muscles and use this information to release build-ups of tension. In the study, the latter group performed better. This suggests that runners benefit from paying attention and relaying accurate information to the brain. Were a similar study conducted in the gym, the results would no doubt be the same – a credible reason for so many exercisers to switch off their iPods and switch on to their workout.

There are other disadvantages to what Professor Frank Pierce Jones, one of the first teachers to conduct scientific research on the Alexander Technique, called 'automatic performance'. The chief of these is that without awareness, things cannot be changed. Socrates, when asked whether it was better to do wrong knowingly or unknowingly, shocked his listeners by replying that it was better to do wrong knowingly. If you know that doing a certain thing is wrong, he explained, you are able to change.

It's important to mention that there is a difference between habits that are developed consciously and those that sneak in when you aren't paying attention. To go back to the car/driver analogy, you will probably have learned to drive by following a series of steps, such as: get in, put on seat belt, put key in ignition, and so on. With experience, you can follow these steps in a state close to unconsciousness, as many of us do on early mornings on the way to work. But, and this is the difference, if you ever found yourself in a different make of car with which you were not familiar, you could, by reviewing the basics, probably figure out how to drive it. If you never went through the process of learning the basics, it would be more difficult. Consciously learned habits are easier to recall and therefore to change.

When it comes to the ways in which we generally conduct ourselves, it is safe to assume that most were not learned consciously. Unless we are in pain or recovering from an injury, we don't think about how we walk, stand or lift something. As the Nike ad says, we 'just do it'. In our culture, these patterns – what we might call 'default programs' – gradually deteriorate. Just observe the default mode for sitting at the computer or in front of the television – it's hardly the stuff of the Greek ideal. The question to be asked is: are we unconsciously reinforcing our 'default programs' in our workouts?

Tai chi

'Grace and smoothness of action in place of jerkiness or abruptness.'

Tai chi is an ancient, health-giving, meditative 'exercise' regime that originated around 1,000 years ago in China. It comprises a sequence of postures, performed with great care and slowness. Breathing is calmed and deepened, distractions evaporate, while a sense of 'centredness' and equanimity develop. It produces strength, energy and self-awareness.

Regular tai chi practice, it has been said, confers the strength of a lumberjack, the pliability of a child and the wisdom of a sage. In other words, it develops mind, body and spirit in a balanced way. The actions are not merely repetitions and it is vital to pay attention to what you are doing or you will certainly lose your way. The interplay of weight shifts, body turns and arm gestures in a smoothly flowing sequence brings about attentive calmness. Muscles are required to act in harmonious interrelationships. Thus tai chi cannot be done automatically but requires wakeful attention – the mind is alert throughout.

Anyone understanding something of Alexander Technique will notice a number of links to tai chi: the central point of balance and upright attitude together with relaxation, the issue of head balance and of free breathing, but most of all the concern for unity of mind, body and spirit.

Alexander Technique operates 'indirectly' – it does not go for an objective quickly and directly, but takes account of general self-management first of all. This requires vigilance to avoid the automatic habits that can lead to tension, contraction, tightening, breath restriction and general interference with our psychophysical balance. In tai chi, almost all postures represent some kind of self-defence strategy, albeit done in immensely slow motion. However, instead of merely blocking the imagined 'attack' directly, the postures very often begin by 'yielding': that is, travelling initially in a very different direction to that which will conclude the posture – the defining self-defence moment of blocking or catching the opponent 'unawares'. This process is an example of how tai chi, like the Alexander Technique, incorporates the principle of 'indirectness'.

The general awareness of mind-body-spirit in action is common to both the Alexander Technique and tai chi. Alexander is more concerned with everyday movements, observing our personal reactions (our habitual psychophysical responses) to life's demands moment by moment. So even rising from a chair or simply sitting may be invested with skill and awareness. Tai chi is an organized, 'choreographed' series of actions that are highly stylized – yet, as with everyday actions, we need to employ our whole self in carrying them out and our psychophysical attitude is fundamental: poise and uprightness rather than collapse, lightness instead of heaviness, grace and smoothness of action in place of jerkiness or abruptness.

Head poise is certainly part of tai chi instruction, as is maintaining an upright body without effort. Unfortunately, the inappropriate and crude image of being suspended from a string is sometimes used in tai chi, which is very unsophisticated compared to the Alexander Technique, yet is seeking the same objective. These and other elements (such as direction of vision) indicate something of a link to the Alexander Technique's primary control of use. Likewise, 'non-doing' and 'means whereby' are tenets that would readily be understood by a tai chi practitioner. Correct sensory appreciation, a core issue of the Alexander Technique, is also strongly developed in the partner-work practices of tai chi despite being related in this context mainly to concerns about self-defence.

Tai chi is a wonderful art but it can be more fully appreciated and enjoyed when underpinned by the Alexander Technique.

Robin Simmons

The exercise bike

'Is it possible to avoid using any muscles which are not needed for the activity itself?'

I use an exercise bike as a 15-minute aerobic warm-up at the start of a gym session, but my thoughts here are also relevant to static bikes employed in group cycling ('spinning') classes.

My starting point for applying the Alexander Technique to any form of exercise is to ask the following question: is it possible to avoid using any muscles which are not needed for the activity itself and avoid wasting energy from excessive tension? In cycling, if the lower back and leg muscles are tight and there is tension in the hip joints, it's probable that the legs will not be able to function to their full ability. Creating freedom in the hips and legs, allowing them to 'spin' unhindered, must be a more efficient way forward.

What is happening in the upper body is also important. Effective breathing is vital if you are to keep going on the bike at a pace that allows your body to operate at an aerobic level rather than pushing your muscles into anaerobic activity. Allowing the shoulders to be wide right across the tops of the arms provides space for the lungs to work properly, also allowing the sternum and ribs to move freely in the breathing action.

One way of helping the shoulders stay open is to maintain a distance between the elbows, not allowing them to collapse, while keeping the wrists loose (but not floppy). This creates more space under the armpits, encouraging the shoulders to open. Keeping the neck free of tension and the back long and straight, rather than scrunching the upper back and/or collapsing the lower back, completes the improvement. Having the bike next to a mirror is a very good way to see exactly what you are doing. You may find it is not what you think you are doing!

I have also experimented with how much of my weight is supported on the handlebars by my arms, wrists and hands. Shifting most of my

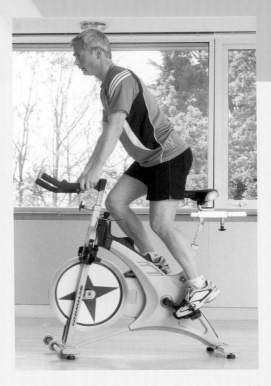

bodyweight down into my sit-bones frees my upper back, neck and arms, and reduces the cause of tension which can make me feel tired more quickly if left unattended to. This shifting of the weight also helps to separate the action of the legs from the lower back and frees up the leg action by removing the job of supporting the bodyweight, allowing the leg muscles to put all their effort into turning the pedals.

In summary, the practices which I have found help me make the most efficient use of an exercise bike are:

Above Excellent use on a static bike, with the head leading and the body following.

- Keeping my weight in the sit-bones to allow freedom in the hip sockets and a separation while maintaining the connection between lower back and legs.
- Keeping my elbows apart and maintaining an outward rotation of my shoulders to give width across the upper chest. This allows greater movement of the sternum and ribs to free up my breathing.
- Maintaining a straight back so that it does not collapse, hold tension or get too involved in what my legs are doing. This also involves using the postural muscles in my back to hold myself in position, rather than getting them involved in the pedalling movement.
- Making sure the bike set-up allows me enough room between saddle, handlebars and pedals, and that the handlebars are wide enough. Too short a distance between saddle, handlebars and/or pedals results in a shortening and compression of the spine.

Erica Donnison

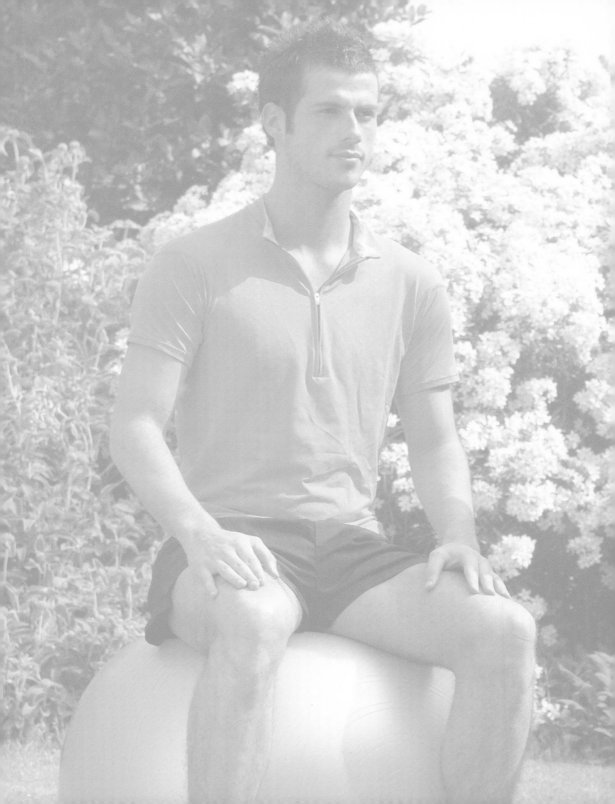

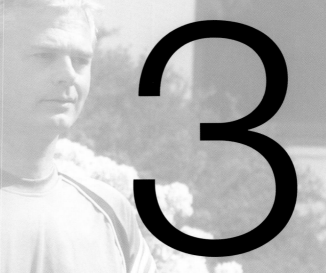

3

FIT FOR LIFE

'I've always said that exercise is a short cut to the cemetery.'

John Mortimer, *Rumpole of the Bailey*

Do we automatically switch to our 'default program' whenever we step into the gym or an exercise class? Let's take a tour of a typical fitness club and find out.

It is Monday lunchtime, somewhere in the Western world. This is always the busiest time of the week as members guiltily try to forget their Saturday night excesses, and a queue is building up at the reception desk. Harassed expressions and anxious glances at the clock reveal the fact that a popular class starts in five minutes – and all the places might be taken.

In the large studio, a circuit-training session is underway with press-ups, sit-ups, squat-thrusts, skipping and shuttle runs. These old-fashioned exercises traditionally loved by Army physical training instructors and loathed by raw recruits have never lost their popularity, particularly among men. And with good reason: most people know how to perform them, they're not complicated, and they address all the main components of fitness – cardiovascular efficiency, muscular strength and endurance, flexibility and motor skills such as balance, agility, power and speed.

Over in the dance studio, it's mainly women taking part in 'Cardio Blast'. To the accompaniment of loud, rhythmic music, funky moves are being laid down: choreographed turns, mambo steps and cha-cha-chas interspersed with high-energy sprints and star jumps. Ever since the *Jane Fonda Workout Book* grapevined its way to success on both sides of the Atlantic in 1981, exercise to music has continually reinvented itself and the basic concept of 'aerobics' has retained its popularity.

In the smaller studio next door, the atmosphere is altogether calmer. There's an equal mix between the sexes in the 'Core Stability' workout, performing lunges, tricep dips, shoulder presses and abdominal curls with the aid of large, inflated gym balls. The ideas behind the class are nothing new, since physiotherapists, dancers and Pilates teachers have long understood the importance of working the deep stabilizing muscles around the spine, trunk and abdomen. After all, they play a key role in everyday movements such as standing, sitting, bending and lifting, and in developing good posture. Here, the participants are learning to locate and engage these muscles with focused, precise exercises – while trying to remain stable on the ball. Little wonder that there's a look of intense concentration on everyone's face.

There's music coming from the free weights area as well. But instead of the usual hard-core crew humping huge lumps of metal around, the room has been taken over for synchronized squats, dead lifts, upright rows and chest presses. It's a 'Sleek Physique' session, and the weights are relatively light because there are multiple repetitions of each exercise: the aim is to increase muscular endurance and develop tone rather than bulk. After all, strength training should be a key component of every exerciser's programme, but women in particular can feel intimidated by the testosterone-fuelled atmosphere that often oozes from such places. Not so here, where both sexes are also getting to grips with compound moves such as the clean and press.

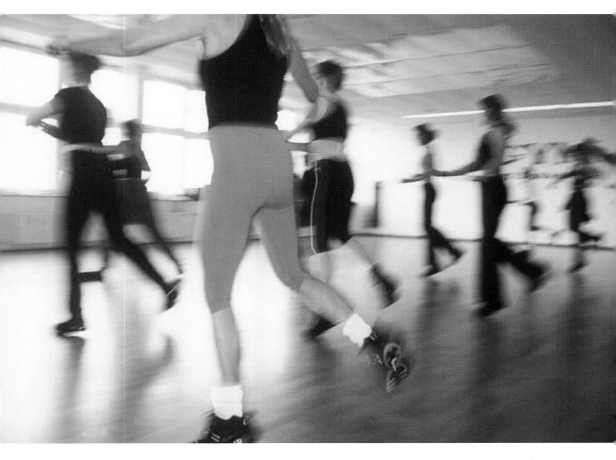

Finally, there's the busiest place of all – the 'cardio theatre', with its ranks of rowers, steppers, skywalkers, stairclimbers and exercise bikes all facing a wall of TV and video screens. Despite its popularity, this is actually one of the quietest parts of the club. Almost everyone is wearing headsets tuned to their favourite channel, while the mechanical hum of the machines drowns out the sound of feet on treadmills. Others grab their personalized workout cards and move across to the weights machines, keying in the data that enable the

Above The high-energy environment of an exercise to music class can sometimes blind participants to the need to pay attention to their use.

equipment's mini-computers to calibrate the necessary load. Eight reps, rest, eight reps again, then grab the schedule and move on.

Our quick tour of the club would seem to suggest that all those here are doing nothing but good for themselves, reaping the benefits of a workout and enjoying the endorphin high that can last for hours afterwards. Now, though, let's retrace our steps and look at what's going on with a more critical eye.

At the reception desk, the mood is actually one of impatience as club members panic that their regular class may be full. Even worse, their favourite position in the room might be occupied by someone else! Instead of preparing calmly and methodically for the activity ahead, they're working themselves into a state of stressful agitation.

Meanwhile, the circuits session may be designed for all abilities, but some of the participants are more able than the rest. Soon, many of the press-ups have turned into belly flops, while the shuttle runs have become head-down trudges. There's no let-up from the instructor, though, as he barks at the class to maintain the relentless pace. A few switch easily from station to station, each one-minute routine posing a new physical challenge. Others, however, are by now dragging themselves round the circuit and fighting a losing battle with their bodies to perform even basic moves.

'Cardio Blast', too, has reached a point where the choreography is starting to defeat some of those taking part. While the regulars know all the moves – indeed, there's a glazed, far-away expression on the faces of a couple of devotees at the front, who could probably tackle the routines perfectly in their sleep – a few are getting lost amid the constant directional turns. One woman heads left when everyone else goes right, while a guy at the back is almost rooted to the spot for fear of making a mistake and looking foolish. Then,

'just to finish you all off', as the instructor puts it, the music is cranked up louder and faster. Even the experts struggle to complete the steps in time.

The pace has been less frenetic in 'Core Stability'. Here, the emphasis has been on linking mind as well as body with exercises that require thought and application. When the teacher mentions posture, everyone suddenly sits up straight and studies the line of their spine in the mirror. But after a while, many in the class have reverted to an unthinking slump. Between moves, they sit with rounded back, hunched shoulders and head thrust forward.

Throughout the 'Sleek Physique' workout, the teacher has emphasized the need for good technique and a safety-conscious approach while lifting. Yet her own demonstrations lack polish: at the completion of every squat, she stands up, thrusts her hips forward and pushes her spine out of alignment. In modelling the bicep curl, her knees are locked, buttocks clenched and neck tight. Not surprisingly, few of her class members are genuinely paying attention to what they're doing. A couple of men are struggling to hoist on to their shoulders a bar that is loaded beyond their capabilities, while several women are using a weight that is far too light to deliver a training effect. Each routine is completed with an echoing thump as the bars are dropped to the floor – 'Let's get rid of the damn things!' – rather than lowered with care and application.

In the 'cardio theatre', there's as much reading and listening to music going on as committed exercising. With books propped

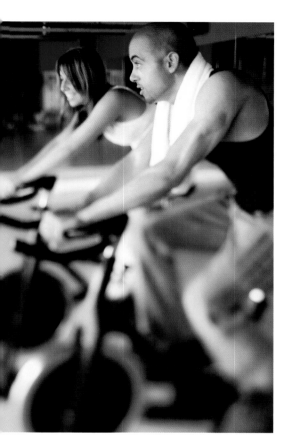

Above The bike, like the computer, can be a strong stimulus for misuse. In the intense physical environment of a group cycling ('spinning') class, note how both participants' necks have 'disappeared'.

against the handles of the bikes, many users are trying to journey into the literary world as a distraction from their 20 minutes of pedal-turning. Some treadmill runners can't stretch the wire from their iPods to the holder on the front of the machine and are forced to run while carrying the device in one hand. Others are stairwalking with their head raised at an acute angle in order to see the TV screen. Very few

are jogging, cycling, rowing or using the weights machines with their focus entirely on the activity itself.

Oh dear, you say. What a dreadful fitness club! No, not dreadful at all – just typical. Visit any gym and you will find a handful of people working out with attention, enjoyment, awareness, grace and poise. The approach of the majority, however, will show none of these enviable characteristics. Attention – or the boredom that comes from doing the same routine week in, week out? Enjoyment – or dragging yourself through a session solely because the doctor said so? Awareness – or slapping on the headphones and switching off? Grace and poise – or just mooching from machine to machine in order to 'get it done'?

It's an inescapable fact that we all operate in the fast lane. It's now hard to imagine a world without email, the Internet and the mobile phone, yet it was only 15 years ago that the comparatively snail-paced fax was still a novelty. What's more, the authors of this book both completed university degrees without the help of a computer!

Such speed is leading us into a life of ever greater extremes, where the impact of global communication and travel – not tomorrow, not this afternoon, now! – forces us into ever longer and more stressful working patterns and dramatically tilts our work-life balance. We may be cash-rich but we're also increasingly time-poor, trying to squeeze jobs, families and countless other commitments into the limited time available, with no space left to relax and regain equilibrium.

Such extreme situations inevitably provoke extreme responses. Guiltily clutching the paunch after yet another snatched junk food lunch, we resolve to get fit and suddenly launch into a concerted bout of gym-going. Yet after only a couple of weeks of intensive treadmill trudging, dragging ourselves even deeper into a spiral of tiredness and anxiety, we wonder why we feel worse than we did before. If we then ask the key question: 'Is this raising the overall quality of my life?', the answer has to be 'No.' And instead of trying to find a more moderate way forward, the inevitable response is to give up.

Is 'fit' healthy?

Just as there is unhealthy inactivity, so is there unhealthy activity. The scenarios in the previous pages are a depressingly common approach to exercise, and help to explain the high drop-out rate at fitness clubs when the New Year willpower wanes. It's an unintelligent attitude that ignores the purpose and process of exercise in favour of an obsession with end results, denying the possibility of finding an approach that satisfies one's whole self in favour of the quick fix. After all, if we feel that something is wrong in our lives, isn't it foolish to try and redress the balance with something that's equally wrong?

For people in their twenties, there may not be much of a difference between being fit – meaning fit to compete – and being healthy. However, the gap quickly begins to widen as we get older. Even though the notorious late-1970s dicta, 'No pain, no gain' and 'Go for the burn', were soon discredited, it's interesting to note that a competitive attitude still permeates some areas of fitness training. For proof, you only need watch a typical circuit class or free weights workout to find participants whose attention is as much on how many reps the person next to them is doing, and instructors happy to collude in this approach.

Models of fitness

Let's be honest: one of the main reasons we work out is to look good. This is especially true if, as we get older, our internal sense of youthful vitality still corresponds to some degree with the exterior bodywork! So off we go for a spot of cardio, some work on the weights machines and a gym ball session to stop those abs sliding over the waistband.

There's no doubt that working out regularly can improve physical appearance. However, we need to understand that some exercises play a part in distorting our frame. For example, abdominal crunches encourage the stomach muscles to tighten, thereby shortening a person along the front of their body. The result could be described as 'slumping with attitude'. Alternatively, overworking the chest can produce beautifully rounded shoulders. Do we really need help to develop these? How about pumping the biceps too much with excessive strength training, giving permanently bent arms that are reminiscent of a cowboy reaching for his gun? The list goes on and on.

What's more, there's a general perception that rock-hard muscles represent the ultimate in strength. In fact, the opposite is true. Tension

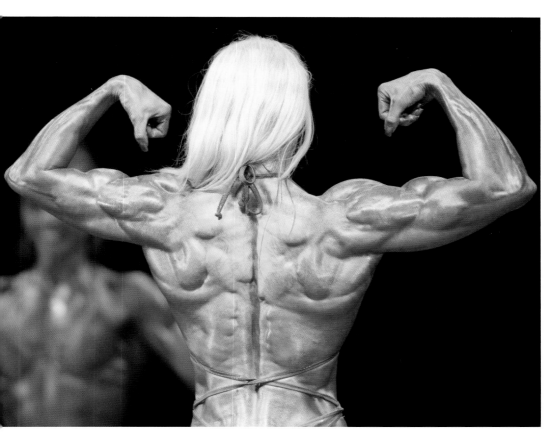

Above Whatever your taste may be as far as 'ideal form' is concerned, keen observers will note the muscular imbalance in this bodybuilder. She is twisted to the right in spite of efforts to develop her body symmetrically.

is not strength. Neither is stiffness. The muscle that is supple and elastic is the one that is most capable of performing effective work. A body packed with solid lumps of muscle may look impressive but will almost certainly be too rigid to work efficiently.

At the absolute extreme of this tendency is the 'con-bod' syndrome, best observed at the fenced-in outdoor gyms of Muscle Beach in southern California. Here are men who have developed their bodies, particularly the musculature of their chests and arms, to an extraordinary degree. However, their Popeye-like torsos are often in remarkable disproportion to their legs and hips. It's as if they have suffered a disease that has caused their legs to atrophy and shrink, looking as though they've just come out of a plaster cast. This contrast is not due to any illness but to an imbalanced training regime that creates a cartoon-like effect by overemphasizing certain parts of the body and neglecting others.

By learning to re-establish the body's natural hierarchy, we less obsessed individuals have the basis for 'looking good'. Not everyone can benefit from long legs, a tiny waist or broad shoulders: some things are just out of our control. But we can all make the most of what we've got.

You and your body: civil war or poetry in motion?

Many sportspeople talk of being 'in the zone', when body and mind are in perfect connection and a great performance flows effortlessly. Jockeys, too, describe moments when it seems like they and their mount are as one and the rider's wishes are immediately sensed and responded to by the animal. Driving, tennis, archery, skiing and golf are among the other activities that have been explored in this inspiring way.

Sometimes, however, a belief in one's own unity of body and mind can be given a severe jolt. Malcolm will never forget the time he took a group of kids from a London youth club on a pony trekking expedition in Wales: 'I was given what I took to be an intelligent animal called Ernst. But no matter what I did, Ernst ignored me and carried on walking after the lead pony. Yelling, kicking and pleading did nothing to improve matters. This joyless arrangement culminated in Ernst taking me under a tree branch which he cleared easily but which caused me, much to the delight of the lads, to be knocked to the ground as it hit me in the chest. I was very glad to return to base and bid Ernst farewell. To rub salt into the wound of my bruised ego and bum, many of the youths (to whom I was supposed to provide some sort of example) seemed to have a wonderful rapport with their mounts and could coax them into changing direction or gait with little or no effort.'

There's a lesson to be learned here, since this incident is like the relationship some of us have with exercise. It begs the question about whether there is a way to improve our relationship with, and ultimately the functioning of, our selves. Are willpower and regular workouts enough to bring about change – or is something else required?

The 'smart' approach to exercise

In October 2002, *The Times* ran a feature entitled 'A day in the life of an exercise bike', in which the 25 people who used a particular machine in a south London fitness club were interviewed about their motivations and goals. All were reasonably regular attenders and their attitude to working out was generally favourable: 'I love it'; 'If I don't come I get really depressed'; 'Love it once I'm here'; 'I tell myself off for not coming more often.' However, their responses when asked about 'cycling thoughts' were also of a type: 'I usually switch off'; 'My mind goes totally blank'; 'I think what the hell are we all doing?'; 'What's next on MTV?'; 'Without TV, magazines and books I'd be bored'; 'Anything but the pain'; 'I usually blank out.' In fact, not one of the 25 mentioned paying attention to the activity they were performing – which is revealed by the hunched shoulders and tight necks in the accompanying photographs. Even though all claimed to enjoy using the gym and recognized the physical benefits, their minds were elsewhere – or nowhere at all.

These participants, keen enough to visit their club regularly but clearly lacking the focus needed to exercise with purpose, would have

Below There's nothing like the challenge of a good video game to cause even the most well-intentioned exerciser to lapse into an unthinking slump.

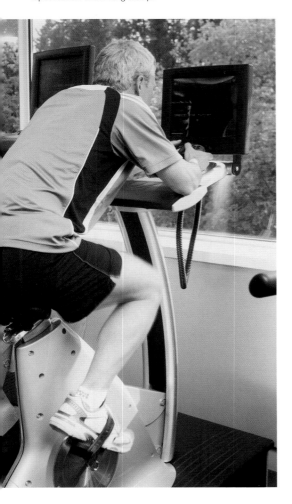

benefited from the 'SMART' approach as a way to prevent the wrong things from happening right from the start – the key to working out successfully, effectively and enjoyably:

S = Skilful: Think back to those taking part in the circuit-training class during our club tour earlier: shuffling between stations like prisoners on a death march in some Second World War movie, 'poetry in motion' was not the first thing that came to mind. The idea that one can perform any activity with skill, grace and courage was sorely lacking in this group. While your fitness level will obviously play a role in how you 'perform', it is not the only – or even the primary – reason for the dismal form displayed in most gyms.

John Jerome, in his book *The Elements of Effort*, describes this poignantly: 'One reason we have pets is for the enjoyment of being surrounded by such great, natural athletes. (Compared to an ordinary house cat, Mikhail Baryshnikov is a stumblebum.) On a recent morning, though, I noticed that the older dog, Molly, was a little tentative, not moving very well. She did a surprisingly bad job of leaping over a small brook – and then I, following, did a bad job of it too. It made me realize that I was moving all hunched up, unsure, tense. I wasn't warmed up yet but that was no excuse. What I was really seeing was that Molly was moving like an old dog and that I was moving like an old man. Stop it, I told myself. Stop running like a doddering old gaffer. I managed to do it for 50 yards or so, but then my shoulders were up around my ears again. I have a terrible time remembering to stay loose, but then I'm not much of an athlete.'

It's interesting to note that in the class we observed earlier, the instructor's mock-threatening tone seemed to make the use of the participants worse – even in jest, any pretence of good form went out of the window in a frantic scramble to 'beat the clock'.

One has to wonder what kind of internal voice this experience encourages in those who submit themselves to it on a regular basis. It is hardly conducive to moving in a free, flowing manner. What is the long-term benefit except for an increase in stress and anxiety, and a decrease in skill? With more reluctant exercisers seeking any excuse to give up, this kind of approach may unwittingly provide it.

M = Mindful: When you lift a weight, do you focus solely on the part of the body that's doing the work? Or are you aware of the way that lifting the weight is affecting the rest of you? Are you stiffening your neck, clenching your teeth, over-gripping the bar, distorting your back, holding your breath? Are you still in contact with what's going on around you, or have you blinded yourself to your environment? Do you know what the proper technique is for what you're doing and do you employ it? Are you interested in what you're doing or are you off floating in the ozone somewhere? And finally, the bottom line – do you lift smoothly or do you tend to jerk, yank and shove the weight (anything to complete the damn rep!), especially when you start to become fatigued?

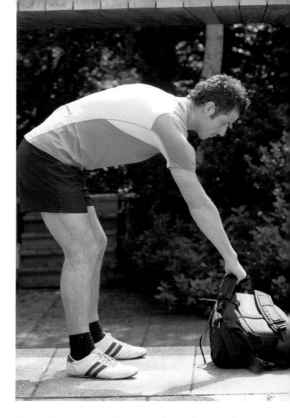

Above Bending is part of many exercise routines, yet does not seem to travel well outside the gym door. This typical (automatic) way of picking up a bag reveals locked legs, an overloaded back and the risk of neck strain.

A = Athletic: Here are two stereotypes in a typical group free weights class: the bloke who muscles his way through every routine with an overloaded bar, regardless of how this is affecting his overall use and unwilling to take advice from the instructor; and the woman who employs such light weights and performs the exercises so timidly that it's unlikely the process is having any benefit whatsoever.

One doesn't have to be born with the genetic make-up of an athlete to start acting like one. In contrast, even someone with physical talents can start to look like that 'doddering old gaffer' with poor use, their athletic ability totally hidden when slouched in a chair or standing casually with hips thrust forward, lower back arched and neck tight. But when the head leads and the body follows in an energized and coordinated manner, simple movements like bending to pick something up, getting out of a chair, climbing stairs or lifting a child can take on the grace, skill, power and coordination of more 'athletic' activities.

R = Recreational: 'Recreation' is defined in the dictionary as 'refreshment of one's mind or body after labour through diverting activity: play!'. For so many people, working out has become just another job, something else to tick off on the endless list of things to do. We need

Below Taking time to do it right. Putting weights on a bar doesn't need to be hazardous to your health; kneeling helps to maintain the integrity of the head, neck and back.

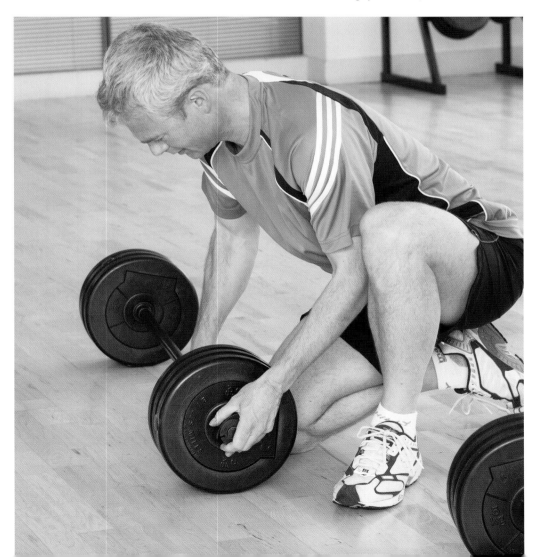

to remember that all-important sense of fun, and keep a sense of perspective about our exercise programmes.

T = Transferable: If we view working out as more than just a means of enhancing the aesthetic (such as developing 'six-pack' abs) and look at its wider applications, then we must include the notion that training should be transferable to our daily existence – what is now termed 'functional fitness'. But here's the rub: many of the movements and routines performed in the gym are not normally found in nature. They are merely creations of the gym environment. For example, when do you ever move your arms in 'real life' in the motion prescribed by the pec-deck? (See p.135 for a fuller discussion of this piece of equipment.)

There is evidence that what we do and how we do it are the limiting factors on what we develop and 'improve'. In other words, performing bicep curls within a 90-degree range of motion only improves strength in that range. Is this what you need to pick up your toddler with less strain? If not, you may be wasting your time. Corrective exercise specialist Paul Chek goes even further when discussing fixed resistance machines, which are a major feature of most gyms: 'They have a negligible effect on improving functional activity. In fact, unless the muscle mass and strength developed on machines is fully integrated through the use of functional exercises, fixed resistance machines will only serve to improve the aesthetics of the body while increasing the likelihood of injury and muscle imbalances'.

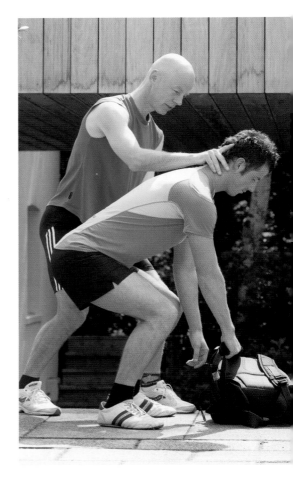

Above Picking up a gym bag, part two: here, the aim is to learn how to 'go up as you go down'.

Finally, if we assume that good use is the gold standard towards which any training programme should aspire, then good use according to the principle of specificity is what should be practised in every workout. Otherwise we run the risk of perfecting – that is, further ingraining – our bad habits rather than cultivating good ones.

WHAT IS FITNESS?

In a purely physical sense, fitness is the ability of the heart, lungs, circulatory system and muscles to function at optimum efficiency. However, this is a very limited definition. As we have seen, we must always consider the transferability of physical activity to daily life. This means asking the question: fit for what?

If you are training for a marathon or a triathlon, your answer will be very different to that of someone who wants to be fit enough to play a team sport, or someone who is recovering from a long spell in hospital after surgery. Fitness is the ability to carry out a given task effectively and safely. For elite sportspeople, that means being ready to compete at the highest level; for the majority of us, it means being fit to live our lives with vigour. As Rodney Cullum and Lesley Mowbray put it in *The YMCA Guide to Exercise to Music*: 'Total fitness includes physical, nutritional, medical, mental, emotional and social fitness. It can be described as the ability to meet the needs of the environment, plus a little in reserve for emergencies.'

All these definitions recognize five basic components:

- Cardiovascular fitness, otherwise known as stamina, endurance or aerobic fitness. This is the efficiency of the heart, lungs and circulatory system.

- Muscular strength, or the ability of a muscle to exert sufficient force to overcome a resistance. By increasing the resistance, the muscle is trained to work more efficiently.
- Muscular endurance, or the ability of muscles to overcome the resistance for a prolonged period of time.
- Flexibility, to lengthen the muscles and increase the range of movement of the joints.
- Motor fitness, which includes such factors as agility, balance, reaction time, coordination, power and speed.

However, the art of working out is to strive for a far higher ideal of fitness than any single element. 'It is a state of being rather than doing,' add Cullum and Mowbray, 'and available to all regardless of skill level, movement quality, body type, sex or any other heredity or environmental influence.' The aim is to live with an enriched quality of life rather than to merely exist. 'If total fitness is your aim, you will have to develop an independence of attitude that makes you self-reliant; you will exercise because you value fitness, not because you are told to exercise.' This independence of thought and a willingness to 'think in activity' are central to the art of working out.

'Gym ball exercises are not about the quantity of repetitions or the difficulty of a position.'

The gym ball has proved a very popular addition to the exercise environment. At any fitness centre you will see it employed to make sit-ups, press-ups and exercises using hand weights 'harder'; however, it is a far more versatile piece of equipment than these limited applications might suggest and has great potential for the development of an awareness of good use. Its aims, in fact, are to promote correct postural alignment together with joint and core stabilization, while improving movement quality, balance, coordination and body awareness. Gym balls come in various sizes: a 55cm (21in) ball is ideal for adults up to 1.8m (6ft) and a 65cm (25in) ball should be used by those who are taller.

The ball presents an unstable surface on which to perform exercises. This enables the stabilization muscles of the 'core' (the area around the trunk from the ribcage to the pelvis, plus the shoulder girdle) to 'switch on', as well as encouraging stabilization of the joints. The deep muscles around the trunk – transversus abdominus, multifidus and internal obliques – are the main stabilization muscles for the spine, therefore training these muscles will promote support for the spine. Research has shown that muscular activity in the abdominals is almost doubled when using a gym ball compared to a flat surface, due to the constant need to maintain stability.

However, before we engage the stabilization muscles or perform any movement, we need first to consider correct postural alignment. Whether we are performing an exercise on the gym ball (or, just as importantly, when we are sitting easily and without tension at a desk), any movement will challenge the body's ability to maintain this correct alignment. Only by training these deep muscles to 'switch on' in advance can we be sure that we are maintaining good alignment.

As an exerciser, progression is the key to every training programme. The gym ball should only be introduced to a workout programme when postural alignment can be maintained while performing exercises on a stable surface. In my experience, however, I find that when I am teaching gym ball exercises, many individuals completely forget about balance, control, postural alignment and body awareness; instead, they're more concerned with trying to perform the most advanced movement or getting themselves into an overly challenging position where their muscles shake, eyeballs pop out and faces turn bright red through holding their breath. This is a classic end-gaining approach. As an instructor, I am forced constantly to remind participants that gym ball exercises are not about the quantity of repetitions or the difficulty of a position, but the quality of a movement and the skill demonstrated in performing it.

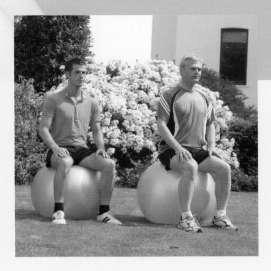

Above The gym ball is a challenge to any exerciser – to maintain direction while attemting to maintain balance.

For effective gym ball training, the following considerations are essential: first, allow the body to find a position of correct postural alignment. When sitting on the gym ball, this will be with the feet hipbone-width apart and toes pointing forward. You should be able to draw a straight line from the hips through the middle of the shoulder and ear. From this position, you should be aiming to achieve a lengthened spine with a relaxed neck and a balanced head. The shoulder blades should not be fixed back, and there should be a natural curve in the spine. Exercises should be performed while paying constant attention to maintaining this position. Only when you can perform around ten repetitions with balance and control should you think about progression.

Clare Canning

An exercise professional's experience

'Mirrors are there as tools to check technique and no one should feel self-conscious about glancing at them regularly.'

A group exercise instructor faces many challenges when trying to improve the technique of class participants. First, it is important to recognize that a teacher may have 30–40 people before her, all with their own idiosyncratic posture and style of movement – as well as myriad reasons for being there. In a one-to-one situation it is usual to give a lot of hands-on correction, but in a class that is simply not possible due to the numbers involved.

Second, it's a fact that people come to aerobics, step or a martial-arts-type class for a sweaty, fun workout with the focus on fat burning, rather than a lecture on posture and exercise technique. The danger of this, of course, is that participants merely spend their time perfecting poor use rather than making any effort to change. However, in slower-paced workouts such as group resistance training or a yoga-type class, it is far easier to encourage people to be more aware of the way they exercise.

Successful teaching to improve technique in a class environment depends, of course, on the skill of the instructor in imparting knowledge and eliciting a positive response. However, it also crucially depends on participants' willingness to learn. Individuals are sometimes unable to take information on board. Some people may believe that their own technique is fine and that teaching points and corrections are aimed at others in the class. Constant reinforcement of instructions and eye contact are useful tools, as is the teacher being available for questions before and after a session.

Despite these obstacles, I firmly believe that it's possible to improve performance in a group environment if instructors learn a range of strategies to convey what is meant by good technique. For example, people respond differently to verbal instructions and may not 'hear' them if they are conveyed in a way that appears to make no sense. Instead of allowing them to switch off, it may be necessary to make the point again using different words or images. As much learning is done visually, it is also imperative that the instructor is an excellent role model in terms of her own performance. It is pretty pointless for the teacher to deliver a list of postural corrections if she has terrible body awareness – the old 'Do as I say, not as I do' syndrome.

Encouraging people to use the mirrors in a studio can be surprisingly difficult, even though this is an immediate source of feedback. In a busy class, those at the back may not be able to see themselves at all – which is a pity as they are often the new or less experienced participants. However, encouraging such people to stand at the front is often fruitless as the issue here becomes one of confidence rather than just competence. Invariably those in the front row are the more advanced exercisers and often, but not always, are more body-aware. The solution is to emphasize that the mirrors are there as tools to check technique and no one should feel self-conscious about glancing at them regularly.

In a slower-paced workout, I always try to draw attention to specific details. For example, when performing a bicep curl I might say: 'Look at yourself in the mirror – are your arms extending fully at the end of each rep, but without locking your elbows?' If there are no mirrors, the emphasis can be placed on how an exercise feels. During an exercise to music class, I might want participants to 'feel light on your feet'.

A conscientious and informed instructor can have a very positive impact on the use displayed in a group exercise class, as well as promoting the enjoyment that comes from sharing in the development of good technique. If this is done well, what has been learned will then be applied to other aspects of those participants' lives.

Brigitte Wrenn

CASE STUDY
Yoga

'Freedom in the joints is not fixing or holding on to them and allowing for the possibility of movement.'

I have been attending a weekly yoga evening class since 1997, and have always been interested in which postures or positions I feel comfortable with and which are more difficult to hold or get into in the first place. After all, different postures suit different body shapes and sizes, so people will find certain postures 'easier' to achieve than others, depending on the relative lengths of their back, legs and arms.

One of the main reasons I started yoga was to keep my back supple, with the aim of reducing a variety of backaches which had plagued me for several years. The same problem brought me to the Alexander Technique, initially as a private pupil of a local teacher but eventually to becoming a trainee teacher. Since concentrating on the Technique more intensively, I have noticed some interesting changes in how I carry out my yoga practice.

Widening across the upper chest and shoulders: Like many people, I have the habit of rolling in my shoulders, holding my neck in a forward position and shortening in the front of my chest and abdomen, making full breathing difficult. In effect, I am 'closing down' to protect the front of my body.

Several yoga poses, such as lying or seated twists, triangle pose and arm postures like the cow-head pose, require an opening across the top of the chest and out across the tops of the arms. I have noticed, both in myself and in other members of my class, that those of us who are closed in across the shoulders tend to end up in a 'pulled in and down' posture. This is easy to see in a lying twist, where the shoulders ideally are both on the floor, but generally one or other of the shoulders is not on the floor at all.

In my Alexander work I have been concentrating on opening and widening across this area and have really noticed the difference. Suddenly, both shoulders are very nearly on the floor at the same time. In addition, I feel much more comfortable in the triangle poses, being able to attain a more vertical position rather than being pulled forward and out of vertical alignment. Allowing time to breathe in the pose helps me release any tension and open up a little more.

Opening up in the front: Following on from this, my next area of thought was to encourage an opening up at the front of my body, to reduce the closing down of my diaphragm and abdomen. Again using the Alexander principle of 'neck free, head forward and up, so that the back can lengthen and widen', I have gradually allowed myself to release the held muscles in this area. The effect on my yoga practice has astonished me.

'Finding the up' in standing balances: Standing balances such as the tree pose have always been a particular challenge for me. My balance has never been that good, so I have wobbled and hopped about for some time. My usual method is to establish some semblance of poise, attempt to get into the posture and then hang on as long as possible, with various muscles doing their best to keep me from falling over. However, what one of my Alexander teachers terms 'finding the up' and then 'resting in the up' helps make the process less one of 'doing' and more of 'allowing'. My 'up' is linked to the idea of the 'up that takes growing plants up'.

For me, carrying out a standing balance now involves being aware of my weight going down into my heels, allowing my neck to be free of tension, imagining freedom in all my postural joints (hips, knees and ankles), while at the same time allowing myself to go up. What I mean by freedom in the joints is not fixing or holding on to them, and allowing for the possibility of movement. A bit of wobbling is to be expected – after all, the pose is that of a two-legged vertebrate standing on one leg, which inevitably is not a stable set-up!

Erica Donnison

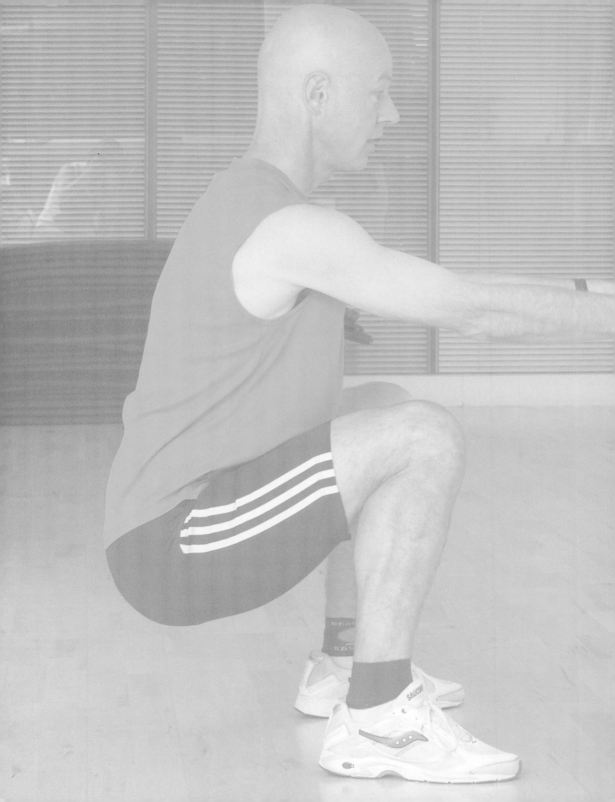

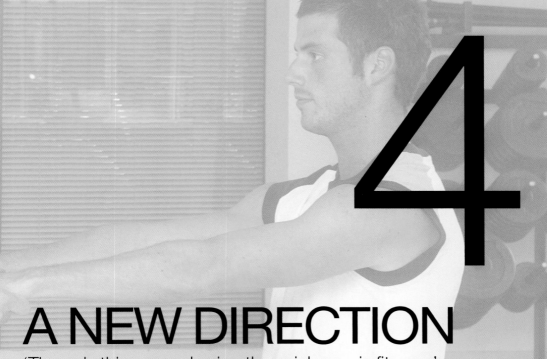

4

A NEW DIRECTION

'The only thing more boring than sickness is fitness.'

Karl Lagerfeld

The visible and invisible in training

When we sit and enjoy a pianist playing the piano, we see someone making various gestures with her hands and body and we hear the results of these movements. What are not visible to the naked eye are the concepts operating within the performer, which enable her to create the music we hear. Two of these are a sense of pulse and a sense of rhythm.

Musicians spend a great deal of time and energy developing these qualities to a level where they operate semi-automatically and invisibly. They blend into the playing, providing the foundation on which the notes ride like corks on the sea. If the sense of pulse (beat) and rhythm were not so well established, the performer would be handicapped in her ability to respond freely to the demands of the music – like trying to speak a foreign language where you emphasize the wrong part of the word.

Clear communication depends on the effort we make to prevent the old and familiar contaminating the new and desired. This requires preparation, practice, rehearsal and awareness. Playing rhythmically or speaking correctly do not demand greater physical effort to be done well. What they need are clarity of intention combined with the means to carry it off. We need to know what we want and what we're doing. The resulting performance will depend on how well these qualities have been mastered. Good technique, whether in music, communication or, by extension, the gym, is invisible. It is only when it is lacking that we become aware of its existence.

The American anatomist and physiologist Professor George Coghill expressed this idea as 'total pattern' against 'partial pattern'. Total pattern is the organization that takes place in a person as a whole when the need for movement arises. Partial pattern refers to reflexes cultivated in response to the environment, 'patterns you acquire through experience with the outside world as you grow and learn to connect with things and people'. The potential for conflict between the partial (learned responses) and the total (innate) increase when the former act antagonistically with regard to the functioning of the whole. In contrast, when partial patterns are in harmony with the total pattern, they facilitate the mechanism of the latter.

Winston, a professional musician whose legs were left permanently damaged by polio, provides an excellent illustration of Coghill's theory. Muscular atrophy has affected the quality of his movement and also his idea of what is actually required to move. For example, getting out of a chair is problematic in that wastage of the quadriceps muscles in one leg and the calf muscles in the other has given Winston the impression that he needs to make a great deal of effort to stand up. He thus creates considerable tension in the act of doing so – not just in his legs but throughout his whole body, including his neck. However, when he is able to prevent his instinctive reactions to the thought of standing up and instead maintains a state of expansion during the movement, the act becomes both easier (takes less effort) and more fluid.

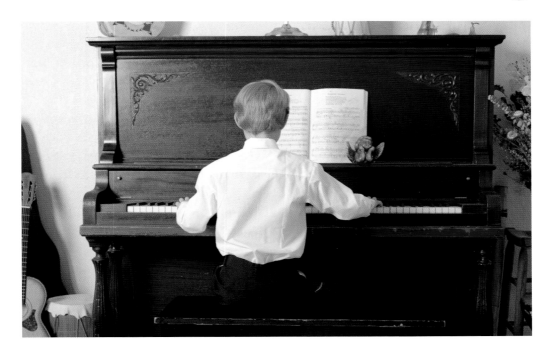

The point of this example is that Winston's legs are in fact strong enough to get him out of a chair, particularly when they work as part of an overall pattern in which his head leads and his body follows. As soon as the latter is compromised, the effort required by his legs to complete the movement increases exponentially – which, of course, confirms Winston's suspicion that his legs are indeed weak and that he needs therefore to push them that much harder.

Inhibition and direction

When Winston is able to prevent his instinctive reactions to the thought of standing up, he is demonstrating a skill called 'inhibition'. This is a decision not to react immediately to a stimulus. It's about taking advantage of the space

Above This young musician demonstrates tremendous poise at the instrument, with the head leading the spine and the arms flowing out of widening shoulders.

between stimulus and response, between when you decide to do something and the moment you put that decision into action.

As we are constantly bombarded with stimuli, it takes awareness and practice to notice what our immediate reactions to them are. For example, a stranger walks up to you holding out a hat. You stiffen and ready yourself to reject his plea for small change, only to realize that he is returning the headgear you had absent-mindedly left on a park bench. Or someone is waiting impatiently to use the leg-press machine after you, and instead of paying attention, you rush and end up pulling a muscle.

Untying our responses from the stimuli that provoke them can open up all kinds of possibilities. Learning to inhibit the old, unwanted response permits a new response to occur unimpeded, which can then be cultivated and explored. Furthermore, inhibition is a skill we need to survive in everyday life: remembering to pause and look both ways before crossing the road can do much to keep us in one piece! The challenge is remembering to remember, so that awareness is there before we act.

When Winston is able to maintain a state of expansion during his movement from sitting to standing, he is demonstrating another skill known as 'direction'. This involves projecting conscious intentions to yourself without actually doing them. 'Directions' can be both preventative – for example, 'Don't lock the knees on this rep' – as well as prescriptive – such as, 'Keep looking ahead while cycling'. Directions are used initially to help establish and maintain overall coordination and therefore focus on the head-neck-back relationship (or 'primary control') that we discussed earlier. They can then be extended to other parts of the body such as the arms and legs.

Let's use the bench press as an example of 'thoughtful activity', where the concepts of inhibition and direction are given a chance to influence the all too familiar.

If your goal is simply to lift a given weight a certain number of times (for example, three sets of ten reps), resistance training can quickly become mechanical and boring – merely a task to be achieved before rushing on to the next

one. However, developing an interest in what you are doing and how you are doing it can elevate any activity into an ongoing process of discovering who you are, a form of 'self-work'. By applying the principles of inhibition and direction, the Alexander Technique helps us learn to recognize and eliminate the self-generated interference that gets in our way.

For most people, the scenario goes like this: get plenty of weight on the bar, especially if there are others around to impress. Pay cursory attention to technique, such as where to place the hands and making sure the feet are firmly grounded, then exhale to push the bar up, inhale to lower it to the chest. Repeat for the prescribed number of reps, with success or failure determined by the ability to complete the set. A bonus might be how easy or difficult the set felt.

Let's take a more thoughtful approach. Let's assume you have a clear idea of why you are doing this exercise, what you hope to gain from it and how to perform it. Now comes the important question: how will this exercise affect your use?

How do I actually get myself on to the bench? Can I maintain freedom and length in my neck or do I tighten and shorten? What happens the moment I reach for the bar? Am I already tightening my neck, shoulders and chest in anticipation of the task ahead? How do I react to lowering the weight and then to pushing it up? What effect does this have on my overall coordination? For example, when I push the weight up, do I tighten my neck and pull my head back? Arch my lower back?

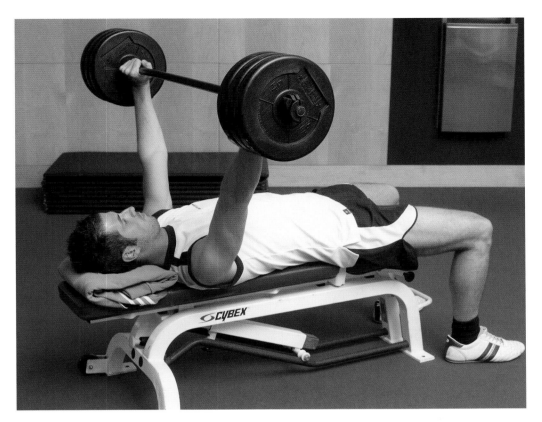

Above The bench press performed with attention to overall use: note the feet on the floor, the lengthened back, and the head-neck relationship maintained with assistance from a well-placed sweatshirt.

Thrust my pelvis upwards? Hold my breath? Compress my spine? Squeeze the bar too tightly? Then what happens on the second rep, and the third? And after the set is complete, how do I get off the bench? Can I do so without shortening my spine in the process?

Decisions, decisions. Bringing this level of attention and awareness will add a whole new dimension to the bench press – or any other exercise.

Non-doing

This term certainly does not mean doing nothing! To understand 'non-doing', let's begin with the concept of 'doing'. This means using muscles in such a way that you employ more effort than the task requires, such as gripping a pencil with the force needed to swing an axe. In the Alexander context, doing implies some sort of interference with the head, neck and back relationship. While we often think of doing in terms of excessive muscular tension, it can also manifest itself as insufficient muscular engagement, or a lack of tone.

In a non-doing approach, the emphasis is

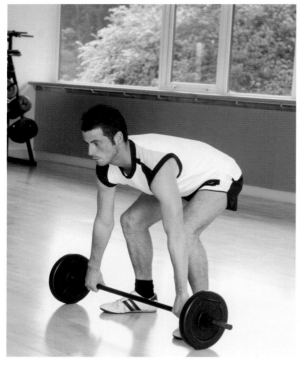

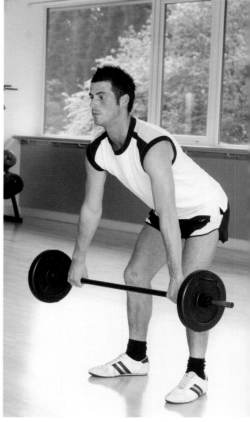

Above, left to right Looking ahead while raising and lowering a weighted bar places a great deal of unnecessary strain on the neck and subsequently into the spine. Rather than leading the spine into length, the contraction of the neck pulls the head down and compresses it.

on using muscles at their maximum length at all times. So contracting is not emphasized and releasing is. When approaching a task such as lifting a weight, instead of anticipating the effort required, consider how much release you can employ to minimize the over-tensioning of the muscles. Use the whole body in the action rather than just a small group of muscles.

Non-doing involves the skill of moving without strain: allowing, rather than imposing. Many of the world's great sportspeople and

dancers, and most small children, provide excellent examples of non-doing in action. Hence the idea of 'less is more' – so long as it's the right kind of less!

That said, non-doing is difficult for us to grasp because Western culture places so much value on doing and on progress. Even our leisure tends to be busy and mindless. The joy of non-doing is that nothing else needs to happen for this moment to be complete. The great American writer Henry David Thoreau said: 'It was morning, and lo, now it is evening, and nothing memorable is accomplished.' For go-getting, progress-oriented people, this is like waving a red flag in front of a bull. But who is to say that this has less merit than a lifetime

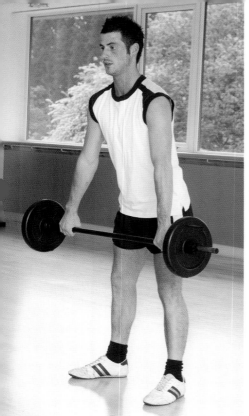

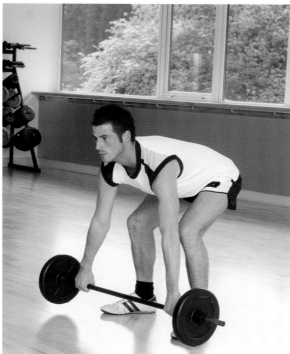

of 'busyness', lived with scant appreciation for stillness and the present moment?

End-gaining

'End-gaining' is the plague of time-challenged modern life. It's the habit of working directly and immediately for goals and results without considering the means employed to achieve them, and failing to ensure that these means don't produce too many harmful by-products. We all end-gain, with our hasty, over-energetic reactions to targets which we feel must be reached as quickly as possible so that we can move on to the next one. Crossing the street before the traffic lights change, we get caught in the middle with cars whizzing by on either

side. Late for an appointment, we guess at the route to take and end up getting lost. In a hurry to get on with a workout, we unthinkingly yank two heavy dumb-bells from the rack and injure a shoulder.

Any fitness club provides a perfect illustration of end-gaining: it's full of people in a hurry to get their workout over and move on to the rest of the day. Not everyone is there for the intrinsic pleasure and challenge of exercising safely and effectively, but for such extrinsic motivations as pleasing a partner or doing what the doctor suggested.

A lack of enjoyment is manifest in the speed at which people complete their routine, and their absence of attention to it. Five minutes

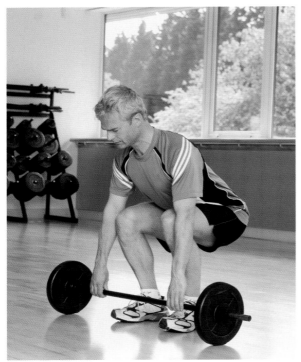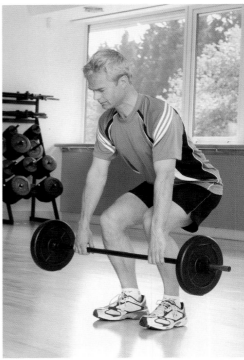

Above, left to right This sequence shows how to pick up and put down a weighted bar without pulling oneself down in the process. Note how the head leads the spine throughout the movement.

faster than last week? That's a bonus! As for good form – forget it. Equipment manufacturers collude in this process by adding on items such as the book rack on the exercise bike and the iPod holder on the treadmill. Then there's the 'cardio theatre', with ranks of cardio machines arranged in front of TV and video screens, which offer distractions to overcome 'the boredom of training', and which further diminish the process.

The 'means whereby'

An end-gaining approach is judged mostly on outcomes: the amount of weight on the bar, the length of time spent pedalling on the exercise bike, the number of kilos of weight lost in six months, and so on. While it is useful to have objective ways of measuring progress, the outcome of any activity is just one indicator of progress. If it is relied on as the only indicator, this can result either in a false sense of accomplishment or a feeling of failure if the expected targets are not met. Albert Einstein captured the essential futility of this approach when he stated: 'Not everything that counts can be counted and not everything that can be counted counts.'

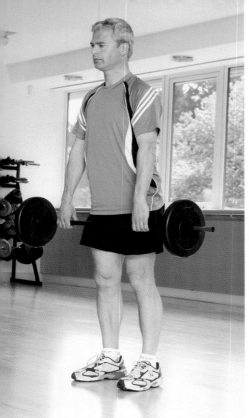
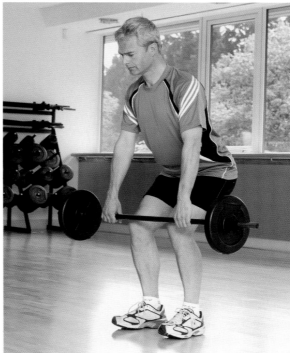

Competitive people often judge success by end-gaining standards. However, competitiveness is not a requirement for maintaining or improving fitness. It may well, in fact, make it more difficult to do so. Real progress is more often achieved when competitive urges are mitigated by a greater concentration on the process of an activity – what is known as the 'means whereby'.

Let's look at some examples to highlight the difference. Many people run to stay in shape, and it's indisputable that a half-hour run three or four times a week will bring significant health benefits, particularly in terms of cardiovascular efficiency. However, it's all too easy to move from being a 'fun' runner, where the activity is enjoyed for its own sake, to the more serious version where times and distances become the raison d'être.

The same thing happens in circuit-training classes. For the end-gainer, success is judged by the number of reps that can be completed at each station or how quickly the prescribed number can be carried out. This kind of thinking is invariably encouraged if it's a drill sergeant (aka fitness instructor) leading the session. Among the costs are poor technique, which gets worse with increasing fatigue: heads and necks drop, shoulders are either hunched or slumped, backs arch and collapse, and the jog between stations is reduced to a pathetic shuffle. Awareness and enjoyment are hard to find, as is any connection with 'real life' outside an army boot camp. It's hard to imagine anyone working in the garden or tidying up around the house in such a manner.

As an experiment, a group of exercise professionals were asked to follow a circuit as if they were working out for themselves, with the results captured on video. Even though all those involved were highly qualified and experienced, none was able to maintain what they judged to be good form and avoid doing the things they would tell their clients not to do! Most importantly, they were not aware while doing the circuit that they were guilty of committing technical faux pas, or working too quickly. The pace, strain and high-energy training milieu blinded them to what was really going on.

The second half of the experiment was a little different. All participants were pre-trained on each exercise using principles from the Alexander Technique: chiefly, allow the neck to be free, the head to lift forward and up, the back to lengthen and widen, and the knees to move forward and away. So, for example, when performing a press-up, those involved were made aware if they were exhibiting poor form such as dropping the head and neck, or sticking their butt up in the air. Then came the idea of letting the head lead and the body follow, giving a lengthened spine and freer joints. Each routine was explored and practised in this way.

The circuit was repeated with one caveat: perform any exercise for only as long as you can maintain awareness and form – that is, with

good use. While everyone became calmer, they also became more focused and alert. In the video analysis afterwards, the participants felt their technique had improved, they were more aware of what was going on and were better able to engage the focus area of each routine. Although the exercises were generally performed more slowly and with less weight, there was unanimous agreement that all had enjoyed a 'better' workout.

Finally, to the weights room, where we can tackle the issue of end-gaining and the means whereby from the perspective of need versus want. One doesn't need a car that will go from 0–96 k.p.h. (0–60 mph) in 4.8 seconds, but one might certainly want it. Likewise, most of us do not need 45cm (18in) biceps or the ability to bench-press 130kg (300lb), although it might be desirable if you're partial to locker-room trash-talk.

What, then, do we neither need nor want? Here are a few things: pain in the neck, shoulders and back; excessive curvature and shortening of the spine; less freedom of movement; less skill in movement; less awareness; poor coordination; exaggerated posture. The chances of adopting an end-gaining approach in the weights room increases proportionately as want wins out over need: when that unbridled desire to build a massive chest and six-pack leaves you open to suffering many of the problems on this list.

Right Balance through opposition: leaning backwards when going into simultaneous deep squats, it's still possible to maintain stability with a lengthened spine.

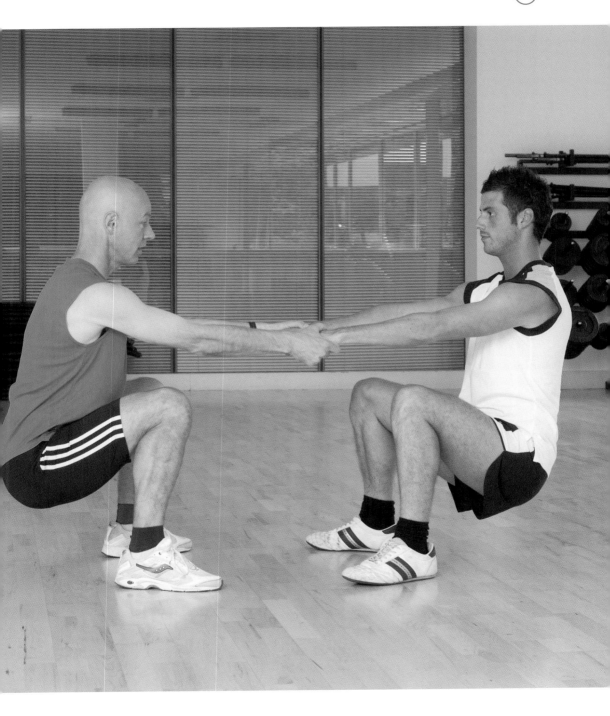

Pilates

'Free yourself into movement!'

From the perspective of an Alexander Technique teacher, much of the Pilates being practised today moves too quickly. Most newcomers benefit from a slower process of learning. At its best, Pilates is mind-body exercise for postural alignment. At worst, it is just another workout.

In my 40s, out of shape from years of sitting at a desk, stressed and recovering from a cervical disc fusion, I suffered what you could describe as a mid-life crisis. I suddenly found myself feeling very old – and it occurred to me that I was too young to feel that way. I researched all of the mind-body disciplines, found myself amazed at the potential for growth and development in the field of human movement, and discovered that I wanted to devote myself to this work.

The Alexander Technique stood out from all of the other disciplines I discovered. It seemed the ideal way to take control of myself. It went way beyond 'bodywork', and my experiences with the Technique were truly transformational. It wasn't long before I signed up for a three-year teacher-training course in Philadelphia.

Over the next few years I did little more than study and develop my proprioceptive and kinaesthetic senses. However, studying the Alexander Technique simultaneously with Pilates (as well as some other movement work), I experienced considerable conflict. From an Alexander viewpoint, Pilates is all about 'end-gaining', working too hard and neglecting the means. Worst of all, many of the Pilates exercises place an inordinate amount of stress on the neck. Most of my Alexander teachers voiced reservations about the process. In Pilates, I sometimes found myself doing exactly what my Alexander teachers warned me about. I pushed to perform exercises that were beyond my ability and completely lost the concept of postural integrity that is central to both Pilates and the

Alexander Technique. My neck would hurt and I would have to see a chiropractor or get a massage just to keep up.

When I tried to slow down in Pilates, the teachers treated me as if I was being lazy. Additionally, Pilates instructors teach 'posture' in a way that would make most Alexander teachers' hair stand on end. Alexander students, after all, do not 'learn posture', they learn to free themselves of unwanted tension, to direct their head to lead and the body to follow and, indirectly, rediscover their own natural ease. Alexander students seem to end up with nicely balanced posture but do not 'pull their shoulders back' or 'stomach in' or 'hold their head up'.

Back on the Pilates training course, I would try to inhibit but there was little time for pausing, noticing what I was doing and redirecting myself in the movement. I just had to get through the course. Definitely end-gaining. On my own, I practised Pilates with the consciousness I was developing in Alexander school. I could take time at home to break down the exercises into their simplest elements, learn to keep undue tension out of my neck and to free myself into movement.

If you plan to study Pilates, I recommend that you take Alexander lessons beforehand and that you continue the Alexander lessons after you begin Pilates. Then you can ask your Alexander teacher to guide and help you to direct yourself in your Pilates education. Look for a Pilates teacher who is qualified to teach matwork as well as all of the equipment. These teachers have the most training and experience. If you can afford it, take private lessons until you have mastered the principles and can perform basic exercises with ease, before you switch to small-group classes. If you don't have access to regular Alexander lessons, even a single workshop will give some idea of what is ultimately possible in the area of 'undoing'. An Alexander teacher's hands can convey a sense of ease, freedom and balance that few of us have experienced since we were children.

Denise McKeever

Olympic lifts

'What was interesting about this process was that my head hurt as much as my muscles.'

We lose around 35 per cent of our muscle mass between the ages of 50 and 70. Combined with the 15 per cent we lose between 35 and 50, these figures have rather unflattering implications…

My Alexander Technique teacher Patrick Macdonald used to say that the two great teachers in life were fear and pain. I think he left one out: vanity. Galvanized into action, I began looking for an answer: resistance training. Something that, aside from the odd press-up or chin-up, I had long been resisting. Continue resisting, I reasoned, and I would risk becoming the invisible man.

The question now became what to do. I knew instantly: learn the Olympic lifts. Not only would these fulfil the requirements of resistance training, but the element of skill involved as well as the romantic notion of getting strong without bulking up really appealed to me.

Olympic lifting consists of two different lifts: the clean and jerk, and the snatch. Rather than focusing on one area of the body, they involve the whole chain – from the legs to the hips, back and arms. They require speed, skill, balance, flexibility and coordination – and strength, of course. Challenging and risky if not performed correctly, these lifts are generally avoided by the general gym-goer. Ah, a bonus: exercise elitism!

Now the problems. My previous attempt at Olympic lifting resulted in a very sore lower back as I did not know the correct technique, but had assumed that the good use developed in my Alexander training would stand me in good stead. So I needed to find a teacher – and was fortunate to find two.

Yatsek, a Polish lifter and massage therapist, agreed, with a bit of a twinkle in his eye, to teach me the basics. He put me on a simple programme designed to reacquaint me with the particular requirements

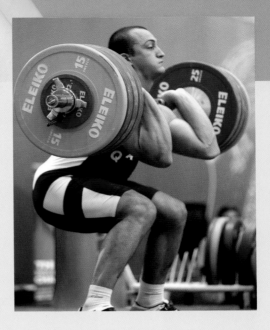

of Olympic lifting. This meant that instead of doing each lift as a whole, I practised parts of them until my body adjusted to the new stimulus. So off I went to practise squats, cleans from above the knees, deadlifts and various other elements.

Yatsek was clear in emphasizing technique over weight. There is always the urge to add another plate or two, just to make it a bit of a challenge. Giving my body, in particular my connective tissue, time to adjust was an ongoing challenge. I just did not want to wait. What was the rush? Why was I in such a hurry? Perhaps it was the gym atmosphere, which evoked in me a subtle but unmistakable sense of needing to prove something, if only to myself.

Above Speed, power and co-ordination are essential for Olympic lifters to manage such heavy weights: a model for lesser mortals.

All went well for a few weeks. No major problems and, apart from a few aches as muscles were required to work differently to how they were used, no injuries. I then went with my family to Cuba for a winter break. I had been expecting to take a week off training as most resort gyms do not have the kind of equipment I had been using, but I was pleasantly surprised to find a couple of Olympic bars and some free weights. As I was practising a few jerks, a short, powerful-looking guy exclaimed: 'Ah, you're a lifter!' While this did my ego a great deal of good, I was quick to inform him that I was only a beginner. 'Fine,' he said, 'we have time to practise while you're here – every day!'

And so began my work with George, a former Cuban Olympic contender capable of hoisting more than twice his bodyweight over his head on both Olympic lifts. To put this in perspective, most reasonably fit people could not even get this much weight one inch off the ground.

I eagerly looked forward to our first session, anticipating that finally (after a long month with light weights) I'd be slapping some real metal on the bar. George took one look at my masterful attempt at a clean and jerk with just the bar and said, 'Hmmm, I'll be right back.' He returned with a broomstick and explained that there was no use trying to lift any sort of weight if you did not understand and employ the correct technique. So that is what I was going to learn – every day!

What was interesting about this process was that my head hurt as much as my muscles. Learning the correct movement required intense focus. As soon as one thing worked, something else didn't. George would demonstrate again and again, repeating, 'See, it's easy.' Each day brought new revelations, another part of the movement which I hadn't noticed. And the practice continued from various depths, ranging from mid-monkey to full squat.

There may be some among you silently thinking, 'What's so hard about lifting a broomstick? I do that around the house once a week and it's no big deal.' Try doing 150 full squats with that bloody broomstick held over your head and your back as vertical as possible (George's was, mine wasn't, which really brought home the whole flexibility issue). The next day you'll want to be wearing slippers or anything else you don't have to bend down and tie!

Looking back on this experience, the amazing thing was that some part of me still wanted to load big weights on the bar, while George, sensing this, kept on saying, 'Not until you get the technique right.' You might think that after 25 years of Alexander training and teaching, my end-gaining monster would be well-tamed and in its cage. If only that were so. The only thing I seem to be getting better at is recognizing when it's lurking around and then it takes a coach or teacher to point it out.

This struggle between what we call end-gaining and what I like to think of as youthful enthusiasm (although at 50 this description's shelf-life has probably expired) is ongoing. As I practised a touch too enthusiastically with the broomstick, my lower back, which is slightly tight at the best of times, started to protest.

After the first visit to the weights room and a few (relatively light in my opinion) squats, it really started to tighten up. Part of me wanted to push through this unwanted setback, which was slowing my meteor-like progress (trouble with this metaphor is that meteors often crash and burn!), and just make my back behave. Another part said, 'Slow down, take a few more weeks to let your back stretch, adjust and get used to the unaccustomed load.'

I knew that the latter was the wisest course of action. However, emotionally it feels like a setback, an unnecessary delay, even a failure, and it requires a fair amount on my part not to ignore the rational, intelligent decision to back off. Perhaps I need to build a fall-back plan into my training so that when I push myself too hard or require more time to get used to a new programme, I then pull out Plan B and follow that until I am ready to resume.

The dilemma I face, like every competitive athlete, is the balance between pushing the envelope in order to improve and knowing when to back off in order to avoid injury. The stronger your commitment to or love for an activity, the harder it is to do the latter. Some people are just more savvy about this than others. I feel that the Alexander Technique at least gives me a fighting chance to find this balance.

Malcolm Balk

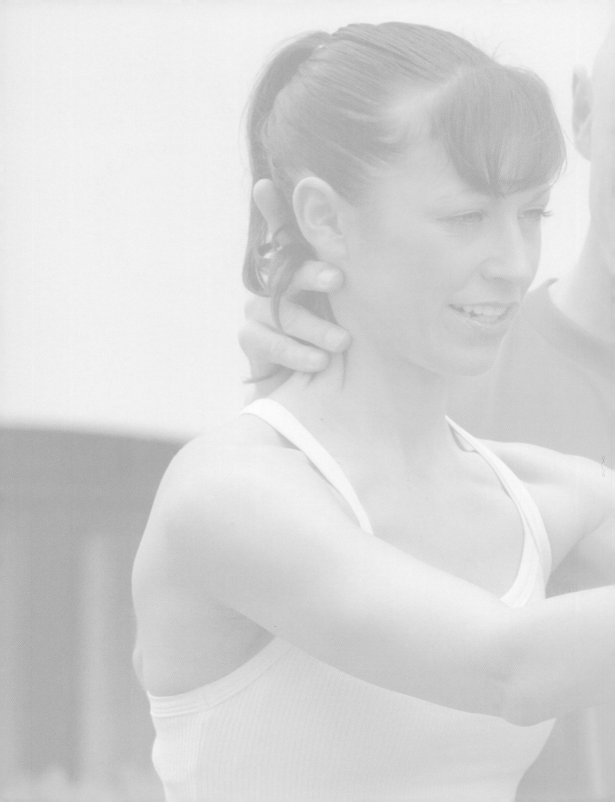

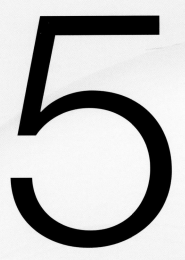

5

THINKING INTO TRAINING

'Experience is not what happens to you, it's what you do with what happens to you.'

Aldous Huxley

When the tone in the neck allows the head to be poised on top of the spine in such a way that the spine is encouraged to lengthen, we function better and move more freely. We need to keep this definition of 'primary control of use' in mind whenever we work out. To help us, we can borrow some of the procedures used in Alexander Technique classes. These help to focus attention on a specific pattern of movement within the context of general coordination while promoting good use – that is, to reduce extraneous movement, misdirected effort and unnecessary tension.

Alexander called these arrangements 'positions of mechanical advantage', which were to encourage a general release and develop freedom and balance. For example, an attitude of standing with the body inclined a little forward, with hip, knee and ankle joints flexed, helps to encourage a lengthening when bending – as opposed to the common tendency to compress and collapse during this activity.

Semi-supine

It may seem strange to consider training by lying down calmly rather than getting up and moving, but ten minutes spent in a semi-supine position can greatly benefit us all. Lie on a firm surface (a mattress or sofa is too soft) in a quiet space with your legs bent, knees pointing towards the ceiling. Rest your hands alongside your lower abdomen with the elbows pointing out to the side. Support your head with a couple of paperback books, to a comfortable height of about 5cm (2in), and keep your eyes open. Here are ten great reasons for lying down once or twice a day:

- **To release unnecessary tension.** A break from the stresses and pressures of everyday living: always a pleasant experience!

- **To reconnect with your body.** Apart from the daily demands of the stomach, bladder and lower intestine (and perhaps the odd nagging injury), we may remain blissfully unaware of our bodies. In the semi-supine position, you can 'wake up' to what is happening with your body, increasing your ability to respond effectively to feedback both from within (sensations) and without (instructions from a coach or personal trainer).

- **To increase balance and coordination.** While some might argue that hardcore gym-goers can be a bit unbalanced anyway, the fact remains that most of us could improve in this area. Try this simple test: stand in front of a mirror with your feet fairly close together. Now lift one knee so that you are standing, stork-like, on one leg. How much have you leaned over to one side? If it is more than a degree or two, this indicates a problem. There should be little or no perceptible shift of weight to the supporting leg. We all possess a set of reflexes that will do their job provided that we do not interfere with them!

One of the most common methods of 'getting in the way' concerns the way we carry our

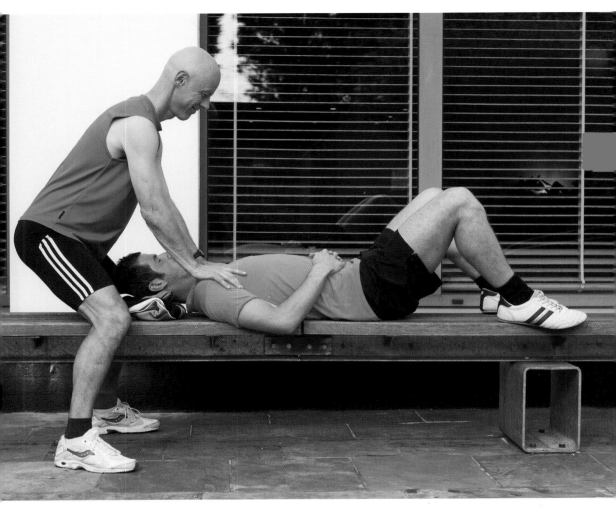

Above Semi-supine can be done on any firm, flat surface and provides a tremendous boost to the recovery process.

head. If we allow the head to remain poised and free on top of the spine, balance is greatly facilitated. But if we pull the head down, we have to work considerably harder to produce the same result. In fact, while a properly poised head weighs around 4.25kg (10lb), if it is poked forward from the base of the neck, its effective weight (that is, what it does to us) increases two, perhaps three times and more. Think about that next time you perform a bicep curl and your head and neck jut forward to 'assist' you on that last rep. Hence the usefulness of semi-supine work. If it is done properly, with care and application, it can help to reduce the way we inadvertently interfere with the poise of the head, thereby eliminating one more obstacle from our path to physical perfection.

- To improve breathing. For many of us, sitting usually involves a degree of collapse. In this state, the ribs end up practically on top of the pelvis, greatly reducing the capacity of the lungs to expand. Breathing then, as a matter of necessity, gets stuck up in the chest and can even require assistance from the shoulders, neck and head (we will breathe any way we can, even if it is extremely inefficient).

Slump in your seat and try to take a deep breath. Now sit up and repeat the process. Breathing deeply is far easier in the second instance. While most exercisers do tend to reduce their habitual slump when they work out, their breathing may still be laboured – and it's not due to the demands of the exercise. Instead, the muscles which pull the ribs down have not fully released and have to be worked against. It's a bit like running in a T-shirt that's a couple of sizes too small. Lying down and encouraging the torso to release into lengthening and widening helps to remove this kind of restriction.

- To give more length. Running coaches advise us to 'run tall', class instructors encourage us to 'stand tall' and gym ball teachers exhort us to 'sit tall', but the sad fact is that most of us don't. We tend either to shorten ourselves or try and overcome the downward pull with a correspondingly

greater pull upwards – which is well nigh impossible. An example of this is the well-meaning advice to imagine pulling your head up with a length of string. Since muscles work by shortening and, in most cases, the muscles in our body are below the head, any muscle shortening will pull the head down. Studies have shown that the average person loses around 1cm (½in) in height between waking up in the morning and going to sleep at night. This is caused by pressure on the spinal discs, plus a tendency to pull down or collapse. This literally squeezes the juice out of our spines. The phenomenon can be lessened if we lie down and learn to lengthen ourselves on a regular basis.

- To improve focus and attention. A good workout is related to what sports psychologists call 'arousal' or 'activation level'. If it is too low, we feel sluggish, tired and unmotivated. If it is too high, we feel stressed, pressured and tense. Most of us know when we are 'in the zone' as we walk to the gym with a purposeful stride, energized, focused and raring to go. Semi-supine can help you become aware of how you are reacting to a workout (for example, shallow breathing, tension in the neck and shoulders, worry about performing well), while creating the conditions for ideal performance (long spine, relaxed breathing, free muscles and a sense of control).

- To move from rest to activity. Semi-supine work can help smooth the transition from a sedentary state to a more active one. Rather than forcing the body to respond to our wishes, we can help it prepare gently and thus reduce the chance of injury. A conventional warm-up prepares the body physically for the work to follow, by increasing the blood flow to the working muscles and allowing a greater release of oxygen to them. However, it invariably pays less attention to mental rehearsal. Semi-supine does not replace an active warm-up but serves as a useful preliminary to it, reminding us that what is often dismissed as 'just a warm-up' can still be approached in a more conscious, coordinated manner.

● To aid recovery. Most of us are not always aware of how we tighten, pull ourselves down (shorten) and distort our structure. Lying down after a workout can help to release unnecessary tension and unwanted postural distortion built up during the session. Left unchecked, these reactions can easily become part of our pattern of use and thus affect other areas of life.

● To boost energy. Very few gym-goers are full-time athletes and can afford to lounge around between workouts watching DVDs or playing computer games! We have to run a business, go to college, bring up a family, and so on. As a result, our energy may be depleted when it comes to training. A quick, non-caffeinated method of rejuvenation is to lie down in the semi-supine position for ten minutes or so.

● To reawaken kinaesthesia. Kinaesthesia is the ability to sense the position, location, orientation and movement of our body and its parts (always a very useful skill in a crowded exercise to music class!). Tense, over-contracted muscles, fixed joints and long periods of inactivity all tend to reduce this sixth sense, and with it our capacity to 'hear the whispers before they turn into screams'.

According to David Garlick, in his book *The Lost Sixth Sense*, 'As a person becomes aware of his/her muscle state, this lays the basis for better functioning of the musculo-skeletal system and will help to prevent or lessen musculo-skeletal problems. Secondly, there is an important effect psychologically in being aware, even if only every now and again, of one's muscles. There develops a sense of individual unity, of being at peace with oneself, of being "centered" in oneself.' Learning to release strongly contracted muscles through semi-supine work helps undo our tendency to suppress sensory inputs and eases us back in touch with ourselves.

Freeing the neck

We have already seen the importance of 'appropriate effort' or non-doing. In one sense, this means the idea of effortlessness, of doing something difficult with no apparent effort or strain. Think of a concert pianist playing a fiendishly challenging piece while showing no more tension than if he were reading the newspaper, or a dancer leaping across the stage with muscles rippling but a look of serene grace on her face.

However, the notion of 'appropriate effort' is also more specific: that work should be spread throughout the body in an equitable fashion. This implies that in order to improve coordination, most people have to allow certain muscles to do less and others to do more.

For example, many of us live our lives with tight shoulders. Yet much of the time we are not even aware that they're tight until we're faced with, say, a piano lesson and we completely stiffen up and can't play the simplest of scales. How, then, to achieve a balance?

No, not by doing tricep extensions after bicep curls, and working the hamstrings after leg extensions. Physical control and coordination actually start in the part of the body where the neck joins the torso. As Wilfred Barlow puts it in *The Alexander Principle*, 'This whole area is a maelstrom of muscular coordination. It is here that those most inadequate evolutionary adaptations – the shoulders and upper arms – will exert their distorting influence during the many activities in which we engage.

'It is here that faulty patterns of breathing throw the muscles of the lower neck and upper ribs into excessive spasm. And it is here that the mechanisms of speech and swallowing require a reasonably good vertebral posture if the oesophagus, trachea and associated vocal structures are to function satisfactorily.

It is close to here that you find vessels and nerves of great importance and complexity – vessels transporting blood to the base of the brain; nerve ganglia affecting breathing, heart rate and blood pressure; nerve roots which, with increasing age, become more and more prone to compression. It is here that 85 per cent of the readers of this book will have arthritis by the time they are 55 (and many of them younger than that). And, finally, it is here that the head itself – the structure that carries man's most important sensory equipment – has to be coordinated at rest and in movement.'

We do everything with the neck. Watch someone perform an action as seemingly simple as standing up from a chair or, in the gym, a bicep curl or shoulder press, and you will invariably see their neck muscles working hard, often pulling the head either back or down. Even bending forward to stretch can present a problem if you decide to look up and watch the instructor. Yet these muscles should not be messed with – they are important sensory nerve inputs, affecting the brain's control of posture and movement. The slightest shift of the head is detected with exquisite sensitivity by the neck muscle receptors, which then influence the muscles of the trunk and limbs to prepare a response to the stimulus.

Remarkably, recent research has shown that the upper neck muscles influence hamstring length and hip flexion: no matter how many flexibility classes you attend, you won't be able to stretch your hamstrings effectively unless you free your neck. Releasing and lengthening the tiny sub-occipital muscles connecting the back of the head to the top of the spine triggers a corresponding release in the hip joint extensor and, in tests, produced almost double the range of movement.

No one would disagree that a strong and flexible back is a good thing to have, but it took Alexander to understand the crucial role played by the neck and head in how well our back functions. Remember how much the head weighs: if we push our neck forward from where it joins the back so that the head is leaning out in front of the body, the effort needed to support it increases several times over. To get a sense of this, notice how much strain the shoulder is under when you extend a 5kg (11lb) dumb-bell from close to your body to arm's length.

When we react to something frightening or to the thought of performing an exercise that we believe requires a lot of effort, the response invariably starts with the neck. You're in the weights room, you've turned away from the equipment rack and are calmly preparing for your next routine when there's an almighty crash just behind you. Naturally, you jump – maybe shriek – and your whole body contracts.

In the 1950s, Frank Pierce Jones, an Alexander Technique teacher and scientist, carried out research on what he called this 'startle pattern'. He used a suddenly slammed door to measure the effects on the body. After wiring up a student to measure both the intensity and the sequence of muscular contraction, he observed that the sequence always started with the neck and head before working its way down through the rest of the body. The implication is this: control the neck and you're halfway to getting a handle on those over-enthusiastic shoulders!

Freeing the arms and legs

The shoulder and hip joints are designed to allow the arms and legs, respectively, to function independently of the torso. This means, for example, that we can lift or swing our arms without having to shorten the spine. One of the qualities we see in great runners is the head remaining still and the back long and dynamic, while the arms and legs move forwards and backwards with grace and efficiency. This quality is no less desirable in an exercise to music or step aerobics class, or in the weights room, where you will frequently see participants tightening their neck and shoulders, shortening their spine and 'collapsing' their body for no reason other than lack of awareness.

An interesting 'test' of independence can be performed in the semi-supine position, with head supported, arms by your side and knees bent. Lift an arm over your head and note whether or not this movement causes any major changes in the neck or back, such as tightening or twisting. Repeat with the other arm, then try the same procedure with the legs. Gently lift your right foot off the floor and then extend the leg so that it ends up stretched out. Most people find a tendency for the back to compensate when they try this. In fact, it should be possible to lift the leg and stretch it without any tightening of the abdomen or rolling of the pelvis.

The benefit of this procedure is to become aware of how we lack independence between the limbs and the torso. However, by learning to reduce it, we should as a result be able to move more freely.

Wall work

Like the floor, a wall can also give great feedback about our use – the way we organize ourselves both at rest and when we move. It can offer an insight into what is really happening when we work out, and provide the knowledge for making improvements.

Often, when people lean against a wall for the first time, they feel as though they are tilting forward. Since we know that a wall is vertical, we can use it to develop a more accurate idea of where 'up' really is, and not where we imagine it is.

Stand with your back to a wall, heels approximately 6cm (2½in) away from it. Now let yourself lean back against the wall and see which part of your body touches it first. If it is your head and/or shoulders, it means that you tend to stand and move with your pelvis pushed forward and shoulders tilting back. If your bottom hits first, it's an indication that you tend to stiffen your ankles and legs and reach for the wall with your posterior.

Ideally, your shoulders and bottom should arrive at the wall at the same time, and the back of your head should not touch at all. If your head is touching, it's a sign that you are tightening your neck and pulling your head back. When people are fatigued and unable to cope with the demands of a tough exercise to music or circuit-training class, you'll often see them pulling their head back into the neck.

You are now standing with your shoulders and bottom (but not your head) touching the wall. You can use the wall to help orient yourself, and think of your back aiming up the

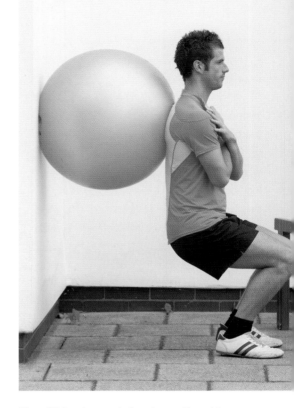

Above Wall work: a gym ball can be used to assist movement as well as to provide feedback during this version of the wall squat.

wall and towards the ceiling ('back and up'). This thought can be repeated several times until the experience registers kinaesthetically and you have a sense of what the words mean. This can be helpful to any gym-goer who glances in the mirror and sees that he tends to lean too far forwards or backwards when he stands, walks or runs.

Once you get a sense of 'back and up', add the following:

Give a thought to releasing the front of the ankle and the back of the knee, and roll your right foot up on to the toe. Did anything change dynamic stability in your head and torso. Now try it faster.

When this procedure is done well, it encompasses many of the elements found in good walking, stepping and running: a long back which tends to stay up and off the legs; a head poised and leading the spine; ankles and knees that are free – giving efficient leg movement, balance, independence and coordination between the top half of the body and the bottom half, with each part working in a synchronized and harmonious manner.

Finally, repeat all this away from the wall! This will increase the demands for balance and freedom, as the wall is no longer there to provide support and feedback.

The wall squat

You can use the wall as a reference for verticality in an exercise which is so often performed badly: the squat. With your hips and shoulders in contact with the wall, think 'back and up', and allow your ankles to release to let your knees go forward and away over your toes. On the upward movement, first soften your ankles, then send your heels down and think 'up'. Slowly return to full height without pulling your knees in. Then see if you can go up on your toes without losing contact with the wall. Allow the heels to find the floor and repeat. This is an excellent way to develop the seemingly impossible: namely the ability to go 'up' (lengthening the spine) while you go 'down' (in space). Also, can you maintain enough length to avoid loading (and possibly straining) the knees?

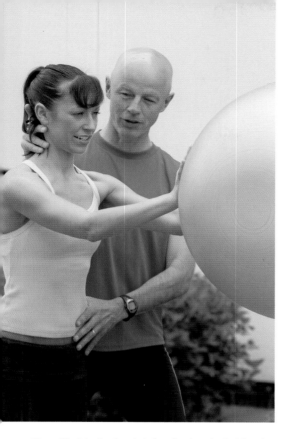

Above The intention here is to lean 'back and up' while using a gym ball to perform a modified press-up.

as far as your back was concerned? For example, did your hips come away from the wall? If so, this indicates that your hip joint is a little 'stuck', and when your leg moved forwards it pulled your hips with it. The other thing that might have happened is that your right hip collapsed and your body sagged. This lateral displacement of the torso is wasteful and costly. If, however, your knee released forwards while your spine continued to aim back and up, then you have the basis of effective and efficient movement. Now try alternating one foot with the other and see if you can maintain a sense of

'Monkey'

Whether in a group exercise class or the weights room, many routines require us to work with our knees bent. This, however, is not something most adults like to do. If you don't think this is true, visualize yourself bending over the sink to wash up or spitting into the bowl after brushing your teeth – for the vast majority of us, there's a strange new joint somewhere in the middle of our back from which we bend, while locking our knees backwards. Other common faults include tightening the neck and contracting the head into the spine, shortening and distorting the back, and pulling the pelvis forward with the legs. It's worth noting that these negative effects extend beyond the legs, where we're likely to focus most of our attention. It's not surprising, then, that we lack practical experience and a clear idea of how to bend in a way that respects our natural design.

A procedure which enables us to lose height without losing length is known as 'Monkey' in Alexander circles because of its obvious resemblance to our primate brothers and sisters. First, inhibition: say no to the idea of bending. Second, direction: think 'up' and allow the knees to release forward and away over the toes. Then pause, renew the intention to lengthen by preventing any tightening of the neck or shortening of the spine, and tilt forward from the hip joints. This should result in bending at the ankles, knees and hips but a sense of lengthening and widening in the back.

Because 'Monkey' is a dynamic movement, it often reveals other postural eccentricities. One in particular is the positioning of the feet:

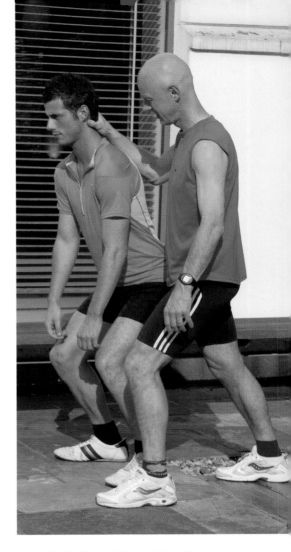

Above 'Monkey' is one of Alexander's 'positions of mechanical advantage'. Here, the aim is to lose height without losing length.

are they symmetrical or is one at 12 o'clock and the other at ten past two? 'Toeing out' slightly makes it easier for the knees to go forward and away without unduly straining the ankles. Contrast this to good use when walking or running, where the toes are better pointing straight ahead.

The lunge

A lunge is like the movement performed by a fencer who is trying to skewer an opponent. The leg in front is bent while the trailing leg is straight. A version taught in many fitness classes has both knees bent at 90 degrees, with the back knee aiming directly towards the ground with the pelvis tucked under. This latter version is sometimes performed with a weighted bar across the shoulders.

Whichever version you choose, this is a move in which you have time to think both before and during the action, so as to prevent misuse. In other words, by moving slowly there's no need to rely on instinct – what feels right – the technique can be practised easily and honed to eliminate unnecessary effort.

Begin by mapping the key joints involved in the movement – in other words, knowing where to send your directions. For example, how many of you thought the knee joint was behind the kneecap? Come on, be honest! In fact, the kneecap lies in front of the thigh bone (femur), while the joint itself is below this. Next, it's important to recognize one of the key reasons for misuse when lunging: a failure to understand that the legs can operate independently from the pelvis. Because we have hip joints, we can move our legs without having to move the back or pelvis.

Now, pay attention to maintaining the relationship between your head, neck and back as you step forward and then, after the foot lands, allow the front knee to bend and release out over the toes. The emphasis is on allowing the head to lead (this is the primary movement)

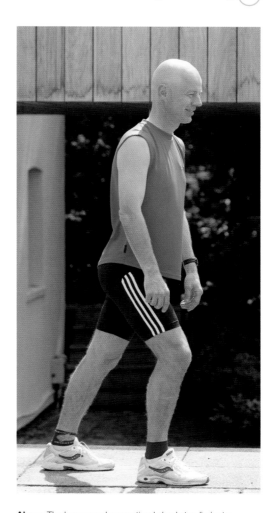

Above The lunge can be practised slowly to eliminate unnecessary effort, making it possible to lean forward without leaning down.

and the leg to bend in response (the secondary movement). This enables the back to lengthen and widen, promotes independence between leg and back, and helps to eliminate the common tendency to accentuate the lumbar curve and tilt the pelvis backward – the technical term for this manoeuvre is 'sticking your bum out'. This pattern of movement will help you to stabilize your body during a lunge without distorting your neck, head, shoulders, back or legs.

Abdominal exercises

Sit-ups and abdominal crunches are popular for a number of reasons/preconceptions. Unfortunately, many of these are faulty. For example, they do not enhance weight loss around the tummy. Nor are they effective at preventing or minimizing back problems.

In fact, crunches interfere with the ability to stand fully erect, as the contracted abdominal muscles drag the front of the ribs down. Gravity then pulls them further down in the direction of displacement, and as a result we recruit muscles at the back of the body to counteract this movement towards collapse. This strains

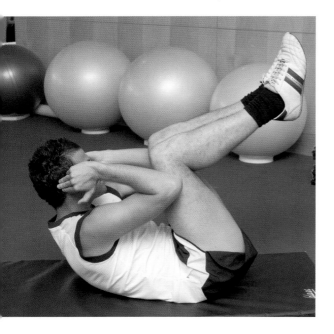

these new muscles that have become involved, such as the extensors of the back, and sets us up for pain and injury.

So if you insist on doing abdominal crunches and sit-ups to tone this area or to improve appearance, it's vital to learn how to do them properly. This involves knowing what's required and, just as important, what isn't!

Let's start with the latter. When many people perform a crunch it's the neck and upper back that get the workout. The head is yanked forward along with the shoulders. This tends to produce shortening and compression into the spine, which is not really the point of the exercise. So the first step in performing a sit-up effectively is to remind yourself what you want to prevent and to monitor yourself during the exercise to make sure it isn't happening.

So what *is* required? You need to activate the abdominal area sufficiently to get it to work more than your current lifestyle demands. However, very little movement of the upper body – just a few centimetres – is needed to provide a very strong stimulus. The correct sequence is that the abs engage in order to move the upper torso, and not the other way around. This way, you know you're working the bits that are meant to be worked.

Left The challenge in abdominal exercises is to engage the relevant muscles without generating excessive tension elsewhere. Here, a conventional crunch position shows that the emphasis on getting the elbows past the knees causes the front of the body to shorten unduly.

Right Placing the hands across the chest removes the tendency to yank the head and neck. However, even here there is visible tension in the neck, which should be eliminated.

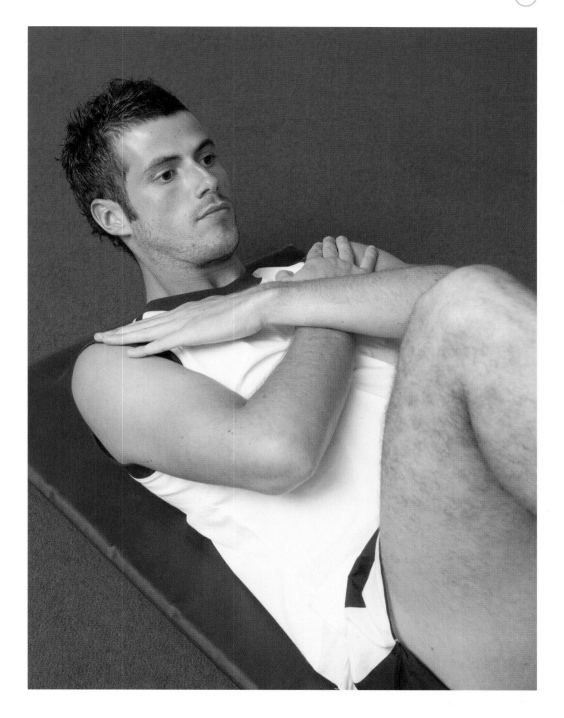

The exercise professional

'Every rep is a performance.'

In my mid-20s I caught the exercise bug in a big way, having completely lost interest at university after the usual mixed experience of competitive sport at school. As well as getting into mountain biking, I started to acquire something of a gym habit, relishing the endorphin rush of pushing myself as hard as I possibly could on the cardiovascular equipment, mainly treadmills and bikes, and on the resistance machines.

As I progressed, I became increasingly focused on the 'end product' of the training, such as completing an interval hill run at a certain punishing speed, or pushing out a particular number of reps on a resistance machine at a given weight. If I didn't achieve those goals, I would be very frustrated; having to take my treadmill speed down by half a kilometre per hour was, for me, a catastrophic failure. On the resistance machines, I would resort to whatever contortions were necessary to force out the last repetition so that I had completed the set.

After about a year of manic training (working all the university beers out of my system!), I decided to take a logical step further, ditch my job, and train to work in the fitness industry. I took a basic fitness instructor course with YMCA Fitness Industry Training, then volunteered my services to the London Central YMCA Club in order to gain experience of teaching both one-to-one sessions and circuit-training classes. Through my voluntary work at the 'Y', I subsequently underwent training in exercise to music, including disciplines such as aerobics, step, studio cycling and studio resistance, as well as exercise for older adults. I loved every minute of it! Eventually, I landed a permanent job there.

As a result of all the courses I had done, my technique had improved massively since my early days of exercise. But in addition to that – and it's difficult to pin down exactly when it happened – I started to experience a change in perspective on my approach to exercise performance.

One element was the general change within the industry towards greater awareness of posture, flexibility and core stability, as witnessed in classes using the gym ball and others drawing from yoga. I completed a course in Pilates matwork, which reinforced this thinking.

Second, I attended one of Malcolm Balk's Art of Running workshops, in which efficiency and technique were the watchwords. This helped me to continue the process of shedding my obsession with the end product of a treadmill workout. Instead, I started to think of the journey through the run as the important thing, using the mirrors to remain aware of my technique.

I began to think of each stride as a repetition, and to judge myself on the stillness of my torso and head, the length and freedom of my neck. This gave my training a whole new area of interest – and, frankly, the shift of focus from the previously all-consuming speed and gradient monitors was something of a liberation.

I hope that I have managed to incorporate these principles into my group teaching, particularly of studio resistance classes. It's important to instil the idea that every rep is a performance. I'm constantly coaxing the class into awareness of what's happening to the head, neck, shoulders and lower back as well as focusing on the muscles that the particular exercise is supposed to be working. A nice technique, I find, is to perform reps to a slow beat, ask participants to show me their best performance in the slow motion, then apply the same control and smoothness to faster-paced reps.

For my own resistance workouts it's the same: I don't worry so much about the final rep tally or weight, but on applying my best technique to each rep, and stopping when I feel I'm about to lose it. It's a fine judgement to make, but at least being aware of it proves that I'm thinking about what I'm doing, not just going through the motions.

Max Bower

The rowing machine

'It's essential to think about good use from the outset.'

As an Alexander Technique teacher, I am very concerned with how people use themselves while they are active. As a rowing coach, my heart sinks when someone comes to learn to row having been to the gym and used a rowing machine to develop their skill. 'I am really fit,' they tell me. 'Yes, but for what exactly?' I silently ask myself.

Quite apart from the issues of differing technique on an indoor rower and on the water, my concern is the common gym approach that measures progress almost exclusively in terms of the numbers generated on the machine's display panel. I actually encourage participants to tape over this panel, save for the figures showing the time spent on the machine and the rating (number of strokes per minute). The resistance, on a scale from one to ten, should be set at about three or four to start with. I also encourage the use of mirrors, and set up a video camera to one side with a TV monitor ahead so pupils can observe themselves during and after a session and note the difference when Alexander thinking is introduced.

To help this thinking process along, I prefer that there's no music blasting away: people become engrossed in it and avoid paying sufficient attention to themselves as a result. If music is a must, then it's vital to choose something that has a connection with the exercise. This means that the music you select for one type of machine may not be suitable for another because the pace and rhythm are different. Better still, use all your senses to connect with your self and your immediate environment.

It's essential to think about good use from the outset. This can slow the initial numerical improvement, but in the longer term is much less likely to cause injury. I begin by asking participants to approach the exercise from a slightly different angle. Rather than thinking that here is something to be conquered, no matter how painfully or blindly, I ask that they try and figure out what elements can be used to support the activity, then free their neck, lengthen and widen, and let themselves move in response to this support. The process then seems to become a lot easier.

As a simple rule of thumb, that support comes from our spine and the points where we make direct contact with our environment. I have coined the phrase, 'Pay gravity its due': this means that if we fail to release to the available support, then the muscles responsible for movement get caught up in trying to maintain postural integrity. Courtesy of our unreliable sensory appreciation (that is, what we think is going on is not necessarily so, and what feels right to us is often quite wrong), this ends up reducing our performance potential while setting us up for excess wear, tear and injury. On a rowing machine, environmental support comes through our seat, our feet and our hands during the power phase of the cycle, as well as through our eyes.

The problem with watching the instruments is that we usually tighten up in some way to do so. Worse still, the display panel is usually below eye level and the stimulus to pull down is almost irresistible. While we slavishly pursue the big figures in an end-gaining way, we set ourselves up for all the things that the Alexander Technique tries to prevent.

To begin with, then, ignore the numbers until you have learned to integrate the principles of the Alexander Technique with the fundamentals of good rowing technique. Having learned how to disregard the numbers, they can then be introduced in order to increase training loads and improve performance.

Patrick Pearson

Right It is vital to consider good use from the outset when using a rowing machine. Rather than viewing the equipment as something to be conquered, no matter how painfully or blindly, take time to think how the activity can be performed with a free neck and a lengthened back. Failing to release to the support provided by the spine, the seat, the feet and the hands can cause the muscles responsible for movement to become caught up in trying to maintain postural integrity.

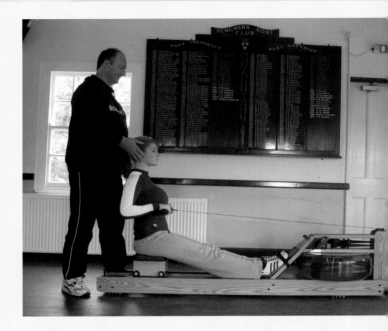

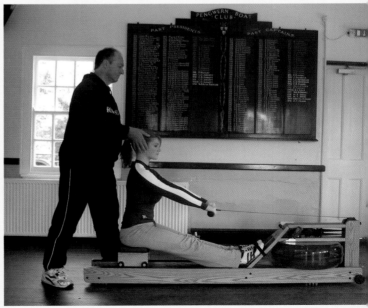

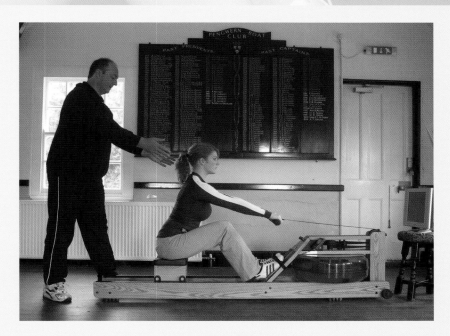

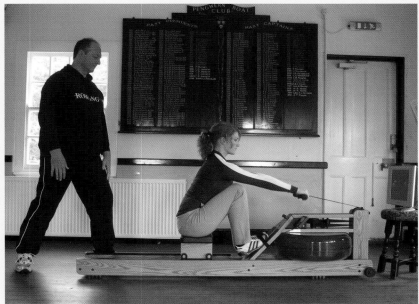

CASE STUDY
Yoga

'By letting go and allowing ... a posture-based yoga practice that was becoming painful to do is again a refuge and place for personal growth.'

As a long-time teacher and student of both dance and yoga, I have steadily been incorporating the main teachings of the Alexander Technique into my yoga practice. I personally have enjoyed considerable success, while my students report similar experiences.

As one example demonstrates, when in straddle forward bend, once the directions are in place I find that the backs of my legs (hamstrings) soften and I can lengthen well beyond my usual limitations. In fact, the crown of my head often reaches the floor without any sense of strain down my back or in the buttocks and legs. Similarly, when employing these directions in the standing bow posture (the dancer), there exists a great sense of freedom and spaciousness in the formation created by the head, back, arms and legs. Constantly coming back to these directions, in addition to mindfully sending messages to energize through the legs to the soles of the feet, helps me sustain a continuous feeling of expansion in my body. Lower back pain is diminishing over time, despite the intensity of my practice and teaching responsibilities. The tightness in my shoulders, due to overly contracted chest muscles, has eased and I have taken on a new and very welcome sense of opening and release.

To my enormous delight and amazement, I find my practice more profound as I am able to work at a much greater intensity than in the past, but with a softness and strength that permeates the flow of postures. I have found that by letting go and allowing, by 'getting out of the way', a posture-based yoga practice that was becoming painful to do is again a refuge and place for personal growth.

Myra David

CASE STUDY
The business coach

'My focus is now on learning rather than on "doing it right".'

I'm a business coach with a strong commitment to personal and organizational development, transformation and learning. One of the core principles of my work is that 'change' is produced out of increased awareness and attention. Human beings are for the most part 'mechanisms' – we have automatic ways of thinking, speaking and acting that have us following rigid patterns of action in our lives. The Alexander Technique pretty much parallels what I do as a coach, not only on the mental level but on the emotional and physical levels as well. The thrust of my work is supporting my clients in being 'self-generating' and 'self-correcting'. It's also the lifelong practice that I've taken on for myself.

Practising the Technique has heightened my awareness in whatever I'm doing. I'm a runner and cyclist; I also work out with weights and enjoy yoga. Rather than striving for an outcome, as I did in the past, I enjoy the process much more. My focus is now on learning rather than on 'doing it right'. This has allowed me to perform with greater ease and efficiency. There's a greater flow to my actions. Because I'm more 'in my body', there's less interference from the automatic thinking that's there for the most part. I'm able to pause and respond with greater frequency. There's a sense of being more present in what I'm doing. I'm more relaxed and at the same time there's a lightness and intentionality to my body.

Fred Horowitz

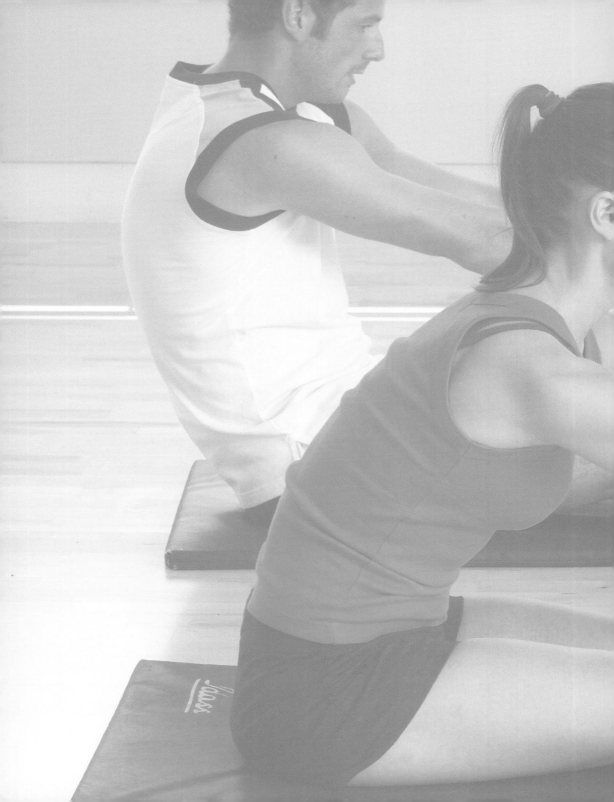

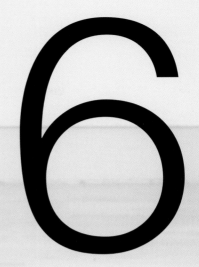

6

BALANCE AND MOVEMENT

'There are safe and dangerous ways of executing virtually every human movement, including sitting, standing and walking.'

Mel Siff

When teaching standards were established for exercise to music in the mid-1980s, a number of moves commonly practised in classes became the subject of considerable debate. An Australian Fitness Leader Network book, entitled *Exercise Danger*, highlighted 30 exercises to avoid. 'We accept that many dynamic sports carry the inherent risk of injury,' wrote the authors, all fitness professionals with a background in physical education, 'and we are culturally willing to take these risks for the pleasure that sport offers. But under no circumstances [their italics] should any dangerous exercises be included in the fitness training programmes of the athlete or the community fitness participant.' Among the exercises on the banned list were:

● The standing straight-leg toe touch, intended as a hamstring stretch but dramatically criticized as 'the world's most dangerous exercise!' and considered to 'cause total body tension rather than relaxation' with the risk of torn hamstrings and back extensor muscles, damaged supporting ligaments and compressed spinal discs. Danger rating? Extreme.

● Straight-leg sit-ups, supposedly employed to strengthen the abdominal muscles but instead working the hip flexor muscles and causing arching of the lumbar spine. Danger rating? Very high.

● Deep knee bends, meant to strengthen the thigh muscles but deemed to exert massive force on the kneecaps and surrounding ligaments, muscles and tendons. Danger rating? Again, very high.

● As for any ballistic movement, forget it. 'All ballistic exercises are potentially dangerous,' the authors insist – and give them an 'extreme' rating for good measure.

This kind of advice was well-meaning and intended to offer very broad, safe exercise parameters for the majority of the population. However, subsequent research has shown that much of it was unduly prescriptive. It dissuaded other exercise professionals from analysing exercises to evaluate the risks and benefits before making any decision about whether to include them in a class. Indeed, the 'thou shalt not' culture can be very powerful: consider that in the USA at one time, American Football players were forbidden to drink water, even when temperatures exceeded 30°C (86°F), because it was feared that they might suffer cramp. (After a number of deaths due to dehydration, this practice was dropped!) Now, in contrast, some people seem to think they're in mortal danger if they so much as walk up a flight of stairs without taking a bottle of water with them.

To approach this notion from another angle, no one in their right mind would think of performing a somersault on a 15cm (6in) beam mounted several feet off the floor, but to a gymnast it's no big deal. Likewise, running 32km (20 miles) a day, every day, would put most of us in a wheelchair, but to marathon

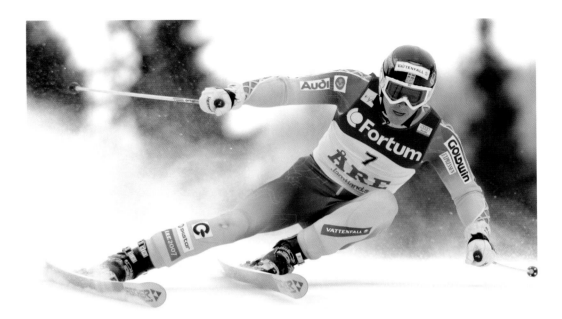

world record-holder Paula Radcliffe, it's all part of regular training.

The point here is that it's not the exercise so much as the individual who is carrying it out that determines whether it is safe or dangerous. Top-flight athletes have injured themselves while getting out of bed in the morning, using a can-opener or climbing into a car; others have ended up in hospital after trying to coax a little white ball into a small cup with nothing more hazardous than a golf club in their hands. So what's the bottom line? If you know what you're doing or, more importantly, how you're going to do it, just about any physical activity is safe.

Interestingly, some of the exercises once given high 'danger ratings' by the Australian Fitness Leader Network have since been rehabilitated. For example, star jumps ('jumping jacks') and burpees – the latter dismissed as 'a

Above It's not the exercise so much as the individual who is carrying it out that determines whether it is safe or dangerous. This belief underpins most of the high-risk strategies performed by elite sportspeople.

definite no-no' – are now staples of most circuit-training classes. The point is that instructors must demonstrate them accurately and try to correct poor technique among participants.

It is, in fact, relatively safe to allow the body to be used imprecisely or inefficiently provided that we work within certain structural parameters. We know that a controlled degree of adaptation will always strengthen the most stressed parts of the body, so long as their mechanical limits are not exceeded. We also know from the principle of gradual progressive overload that this repeated activity will make these stressed structures increasingly strong, so that they will be better equipped to handle poor technique or deviations from the recommended norm. As a result, it's fair to argue that perfect training produces maladaptation, while integrated, well-sequenced phases of perfection and imperfection produce superior functional adaptation.

As for ballistic stretching and its place on the 'banned list', there is now evidence that avoiding ballistic loading may produce tissues that are actually more vulnerable to injury if we're suddenly required to produce a ballistic action in sport or everyday life. Avoiding a particular exercise in training just because it's not recommended by fitness professionals could predispose us to greater danger if we find ourselves having to make such a move on the sports field or while engaged in heavy manual labour.

Such advice can leave us confused about the way to progress our own exercise routines. After all, our aim is to find a balanced approach to working out, just as we want to find balance in today's world, feel at one with ourselves and become better able to interact with our fast-paced and demanding environment.

When balance is addressed in the context of exercise, it's often related to weight training. One needs to balance muscle groups: the prime movers with the antagonists. So if you work your biceps (the prime mover that initiates flexion in an arm curl) you also need to train your triceps (the antagonist muscle which opposes the action of the prime mover), so that a balance can be achieved between the two

groups. From an Alexander perspective, however, it's important to think about balance more generally: at rest, in activity and, in both, between the working and supporting muscles.

Posture imperfect

In Western society, it is sad but true that the slump is much more the norm than the beautifully lengthened back of the tribesman or woman. It's not surprising, then, that at the beginning of any group exercise class you can guarantee the instructor will mention posture. However, this is merely a cue for participants to look at themselves in the mirrors and assume some variation on a military stance: the neck tightened and the head pulled into the spine, causing it to compress, and the chest raised, causing the lower back to tighten and hollow and the knees and legs to stiffen. Such a position actually requires considerable effort to maintain. How can anyone possibly hope to begin moving naturally and efficiently having adopted it?

Advice may follow about the need to develop the abdominal and back muscles to 'stabilize and support' the torso (this is, of course, the basic premise behind the 'core stability' workout developed from the principles of Pilates); sometimes, the recommendation will be to tighten the abdominal muscles and reduce the distance between the belly button and spine. Additional corrective measures may

Right This is a superb example of a 'natural squat'. Note the head leading and the back following, as well as the range of movement in the hips, knees and ankles. Compare this to what is so often seen in the gym.

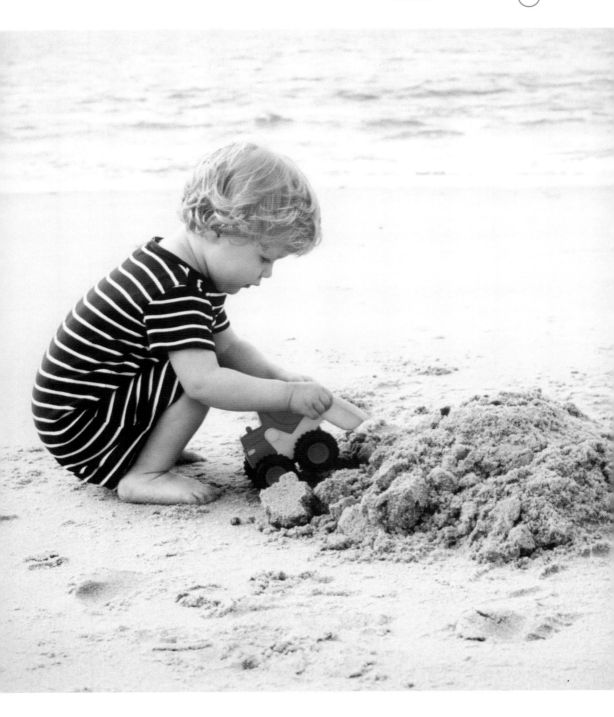

be suggested, including tilting the pelvis and tucking the chin. One of the problems with this approach is that it tends to pull things together: the pelvic tilt pushes the pelvis into the legs and the chin tuck pulls the head into the neck.

A tendency to tighten or fix has at least three negative effects: it makes it harder to breathe, it makes it harder to move, and it makes us less aware of what may be going on in our bodies. It's also based on the premise that more and more needs to be added on. Granted, additional tone and elasticity wouldn't hurt many of us but the main aim is to find out what doesn't need to be there and to stop it. For example, the correction for someone who pushes his head and neck forward is not to start pulling the chin in, but simply to stop pushing the head and neck forward (and not to prevent the pushing forwards by tightening up, either).

Stability in the torso is dynamic in nature, with the head remaining poised on top of the spine and the back tending to lengthen and widen. The result is a state of dynamic stability, characterized by expansion of the whole body framework rather than contraction.

Balanced effort and balance in movement are essential elements in any exercise routine. When they come together in sport, dance or music, extraordinary feats can be achieved. This is the experience often described as being 'in the zone', when the chief aim of the participant is to 'get out of the way and let it happen'. In this state, it is as if the movement 'does' itself: the normal sense of effort is suspended and action simply follows intention.

Does the Alexander Technique offer a guide through this confusion? Yes and no. Alexander felt that if a person is trying to change a pattern of misuse – and we've already seen how, under conditions of increased stress, misuse tends to get worse rather than better – then it seems counterproductive to keep digging when already in a hole. So, for example, if a person tightens his neck, pushes his head forward and strains his spine every time he takes a sip from a cup of tea, it would be pointless and deluded to imagine that regular weight training is going to improve that pattern. In fact, it could well make it worse.

However, there's another view: that life is meant to be lived. Thus, once a person has a basic grasp of what they're up against in terms of habit and has an understanding of how to work on themselves while they're exercising, then the gym provides a marvellous opportunity to test their skills and developing awareness in circumstances outside the normal. What's more, being in a different situation or reacting to a new and stronger stimulus sometimes provides a window of insight that's not always available in the grey background of the familiar. This means that 'working on oneself as one is working out' is among the very best ways to bring balance to the gym.

In the zone

In a typical course of Alexander Technique lessons, a pupil will be given the experience of being 'in the zone' during various procedures. One of these is known as 'chair work'. It isn't meant as an exercise to practise on your own, since it isn't the movement that's important per se, but how one reacts before and during the activity that is of critical importance. We all know how crucial outside feedback is – and for anyone who doubts this, never forget that even the world's best sports stars have a coach.

What's so difficult about standing up and sitting down, you ask? Not much, it might seem – surely most people can improve the biomechanics of this activity fairly quickly. So what does this procedure teach us? Here is a description from a pupil's first lesson:

'My first experience of making a habitual movement without habitual effort seems as vivid to me now as it was when A. R. Alexander (brother of F. M.) demonstrated the movement from sitting to standing in 1938. Alexander made a few slight changes in the way I was sitting (they seemed quite arbitrary to me and I could not remember afterwards what they were) then, asking me to leave my head as it was, he initiated the upward movement without further instruction. Before I had a chance to organize my habitual response, the movement was completed and I found myself standing in a position that felt strangely comfortable. I was fully conscious throughout the movement, and it was a consciousness not of being moved by someone else – Alexander appeared to be making no effort whatever – but by a set of reflexes whose operation I knew nothing about. The most striking aspect of the movement, however, was the sensory effect of lightness that it had induced. The feeling had not been present at the start, nor had it been suggested to me: it was clearly a direct effect of the movement. While it lasted, everything I did, including breathing, became easier – leaving me with the certainty that I had glimpsed a new world of experiences which had more to offer than the limited set of movement patterns, attitudes, and responses to which I was accustomed.'

What Frank Pierce Jones, Alexander Technique teacher and author of *Freedom to Change*, experienced in this lesson would obviously vary from person to person according to the skill and knowledge of the teacher. Nevertheless, it's not at all uncommon for most Alexander pupils and can be applied to the gym by developing a sense of kinaesthetic intuition. It's like an early warning system which allows us to sense when things are veering off course before they go too far wrong. The following sailing analogy, from Ben Wright, can easily be adapted to the variable seas of the modern fitness club:

'The able sailor does not plot, he responds. He sees what's coming by the ripple of the water. He hears what's coming by the whistle of the wind. He feels what's coming on his hair and cheeks before boat or sail respond by heeling over or slacking upright. The able sailor rides the wind, responding without much figuring out, allowing the wind to take him but in the direction he wants to go.'

Like the sailor who depends on feedback both from without and within, the gym-goer exercising with awareness and application will come to rely on two key discoveries:

First, the experience of free, effortless, light movement. Once you get a taste of this, it's like

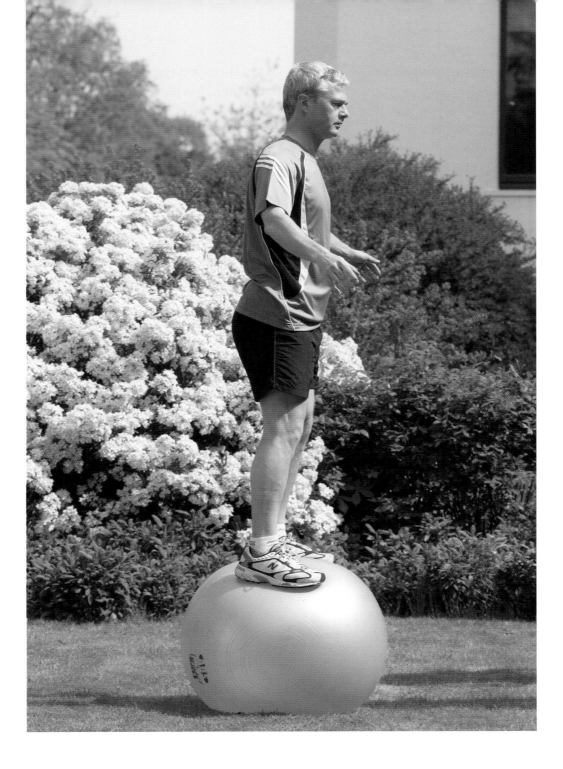

good chocolate – in an emergency you might eat the cheap stuff, but given the choice, you definitely know which you prefer.

Second, the ability to return to a balanced resting state. This gives us the capacity not only to release unnecessary muscular tension before it becomes permanently incorporated into what we think of as ourselves, but also gives us a norm from which we can know when we're slipping off course.

Here are some simple tests that any exerciser can try, to explore their own state of balance or imbalance:

- From a standing position, begin walking forward without 'telegraphing' the foot with which you're going to take your first step. The aim should be to minimize the shifting of all your weight on to the supporting leg.

- Now come to a stop and see how vertically you stand without trying to correct or straighten yourself.

- Lift both your arms above your head as if you were putting an object on a high shelf. Can you do this without leaning backwards or tightening your neck and shoulders?

- With eyes closed and arms by your sides, lift your arms so that they are parallel to the floor. Then open your eyes and, with the help of a mirror, check and see if they are parallel.

Left Even difficult manoeuvres, such as standing on an unstable gym ball, can be performed by focusing on the key components of 'good use'.

Thinking into movement

Forget Jane Fonda's famous phrase, 'No pain, no gain'. For most people, the ultimate fitness mantra is 'No pain, more gain'. Sadly for those who'll try anything to avoid raising their heart rate, becoming fitter requires us to move in some way. This can be either in a cyclical and repetitive manner such as on the treadmill or exercise bike, in short bursts such as when we lift weights, or semi-creatively as in an exercise to music or step class.

Assuming that overcoming inertia – that is, getting off the couch in the first place – is not an issue, the question becomes this: how do you go into motion? Do you lengthen and release, or is it more a case of shorten and shove? And why do we need to bother ourselves about this?

The first answer stems from the notion that everything is connected: that what you do in the gym and, most importantly, how you do it, will be reflected in your 'real' everyday life. This means that while you may be gaining strength or boosting your endurance, your use may actually be becoming worse. For proof, look around and you will see plenty of sportspeople, performers and personal trainers who are extremely fit but who do not use themselves well. Watch a group of dancers slump over a coffee after a tough class, while even the most polished exercise professional will sit cross-legged, mobile phone clamped between ear and shoulder, when not 'on duty'.

In terms of the 'use of ourselves', it's impossible to sit on the fence: we tend either to get better or to get worse. The motion of someone who may once have been a stylish and fluid runner will, over time, degenerate into more of a shuffle than a stride. While most gym-goers pay only lip service to the importance of good form/use when training, faulty sensory awareness combined with an end-gaining attitude wreak havoc with these good intentions. So how can you encourage people to 'think' in a way that is going to change and benefit them?

Initiating movement

In all forms of movement, one of the crucial moments is the transition from stillness to motion, or from one kind of movement to another, as in walking to running. The aim of the 'Zen workout' is to encourage particular attention to this transition stage, helping us learn to 'think in activity' and to inform movement with thought. Though initially designed for walkers and runners, it can be adapted to any form of exercise.

In walking or running, the basic pulse is the notion of lengthening. What needs to be mastered is the free, released movement (bending) of the hip, knee and ankle. The challenge is to maintain length and bend the knee at the same time.

Let's apply this to weight training. First, spend some time directing yourself to 'free the neck' and see what happens when you begin to perform, for example, a slow bicep curl. What changes? Can you keep lengthening – that is, not shorten the neck and spine as you start the movement of the arms? The point to remember is this: what value is it to strengthen

your arms if you contract your neck and compress your spine as well?

After completing the rep, you should re-establish your directions and prepare to notice what happens in the next rep. In each instance, the idea is to use the stationary or slower portion of the cycle to strengthen the sense of good use – to 'inhibit and direct'. Then the aim is to see if this approach can be maintained as the demand of the movement increases, perhaps with a heavier weight, or a longer set, or a quicker tempo.

The following exercise focuses on what happens in the time between the decision to take a step and the moment when you actually take it, and shows how the mere notion of moving a leg affects the rest of the body. Stand a few paces in front of a friend and try to guess with which foot the other person will take a step. You'll almost always get it right. Why? Because we generally telegraph our intention by moving all our weight sideways, dropping it onto one leg then dragging the hip down and out and launching ourselves forward. This habit (along with standing on one leg and, more commonly, sitting with the legs crossed) can lead to what has been called 'lateral pelvic tilt'.

How, then, do we get ourselves moving? Whether it's walking or running, on a treadmill, in an exercise to music class or during circuit training, the first thought must always be to gain your full height. Having established and engaged the conscious directions for this, your

Right This boy runs with a beautiful spiralling action around a lengthened spine and a well-poised head. No wonder he's smiling!

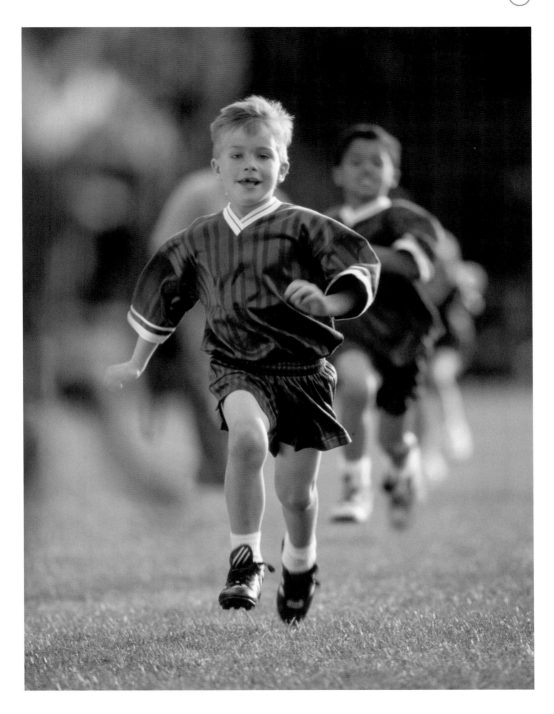

upright body is now at its most precarious position, being fully alive and poised. The very smallest amount of forward inclination will start the process of walking, whereby you find yourself in effect 'falling upwards' as you travel forwards. Simply releasing one ankle and knee and taking a small step will re-establish your support without compromising your length or contributing to lateral pelvic tilt. It's a bit of an art (but fun as well) to find that delicate state of allowing yourself to be slightly out of balance so that you can take advantage of the gentle pull that gravity so generously provides.

Once you're moving, the back needs to remain 'back and up' so that you come up off the legs and the legs can move freely. This might seem simple and obvious, but many of us employ physical tension in such a way that there is a tendency to shorten the spine and legs by pressing down through the floor instead of lightening that pressure by lengthening the body and easing forward and up. We are, in effect, making ourselves heavy.

This view is supported by Pete Egoscue in his book, 'The Egoscue Method of Health Through Motion': 'The symptoms we blame on high-impact aerobics or other sports are really symptoms of lack of proper motion,' he writes. 'A head that is out of its proper design position – forward and down – is a head that makes the neck and upper spine muscles do a job they were not intended to perform. The muscles are there to allow the head to turn left and right; to permit the head to tilt up and down; and to cushion the impact that is transmitted upward through the spinal column and the rest of the

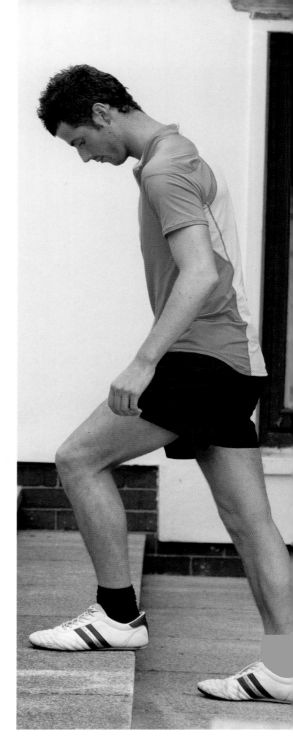

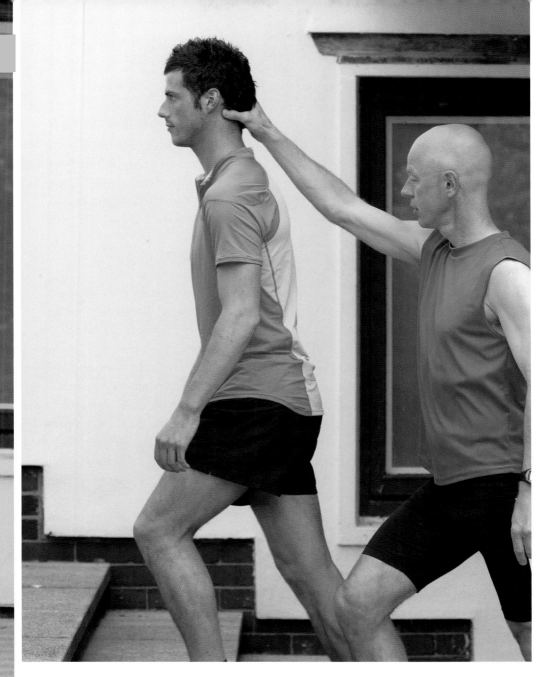

Left Walking up a flight of stairs doesn't have to be such a'down'. The head is a heavy weight balanced at the top of the spinal column and, when it topples forward in this way, gravity affects the rest of the torso.

Above Leading with the head allows the back (and energy) to go up, up, up. By lengthening the body and lightening the pressure exerted on the ground, the legs can move freely and physical tension is reduced.

skeleton when the foot hits the ground. If the head slumps forward, the muscles must prevent gravity from pulling the upper torso over into a foetal position. The head is a heavy weight balanced at the top of the spinal column, and once it starts to topple forward the muscles can do nothing else but struggle mightily to stave off disaster. They lose the ability to function as shock absorbers.'

Walking into running

Everyone is capable of learning to take a first step without collapsing on one side or leaning backwards behind the vertical. The next big challenge is to allow yourself to be in a continuous state of 'controlled imbalance' as you carry on, thus allowing gravity to help with each step. However, all the qualities of good walking lead nicely into good running with only minor adjustments.

Whether indoors or out, first bend at the elbows and tone up the wrists so they don't flop. Rather than trying to initiate the transition with the legs by taking a long first running stride, simply release more (fall from the ankles) and begin to pull the supporting foot off the ground while allowing the landing foot to find its place as lightly as possible. The sense of flow should be like releasing a car into first gear so that the transition from stop to start is imperceptible.

Never be afraid to rest – whether to enjoy the scenery, grab a drink, greet a friend or because you don't feel that you're moving well. Try to iron out any leaping, shoving, lurching or jerking by releasing the neck, lengthening

yourself and seeing how smooth you can make that first step.

The eyes have it

The common habit of looking at the ground when running, walking or cycling has a negative effect on the head-neck-back relationship. But there is a more subtle form of misuse of the eyes and the way we see, which often goes unnoticed.

Anyone who sits typing at a computer may be aware that they are looking either at the screen or at the keyboard with an intense, 'narrow' focus. At other times they may be gazing, unseeing, into space, hoping for inspiration. While both these visual tics have their purpose, seeing in this way habitually encourages a tendency to pull the head forward and thus bring about a reduction in our visual field so that little, if any, of our peripheral vision is used. This cuts us off from ourselves and from our surroundings. Emotionally, there is often a vague sense of anxiety associated with this kind of 'looking'.

The same pattern is often present when we exercise. We either gaze intently at the ground or at some distant target, or we move without registering what our eyes are telling us. Learning to work out with 'receptive eyes' has a marked effect on the quality of the experience. It involves becoming aware of this tendency to focus on a small part of the visual field, then allowing more of what is in front of us to register passively with the eyes but actively in terms of awareness – in other words, beginning to 'see what we are looking at'. Because we aren't seeking out with the eyes, the neck can soften and stop pulling the head forward. Allowing ourselves to see not just what is immediately in front of us, but also the wider view, activates our peripheral vision and makes us more aware of what is going on within.

In her excellent book on horseriding, *Body Sense*, Sally Tottle points out that riding with 'receptive eyes' helps the rider become more aware of her seat, the most important link between horse and rider. Running or performing an exercise to music class with receptive eyes will provide a connection with the feet and greater awareness of your contact with the ground, such as a soft or hard landing, and whether you are landing on the ball of the foot or the heel.

Without and within

By widening our contact with the outside world in this way, we often find ourselves more accurately connecting with what is happening internally. In the gym, an idea to explore could be weight training – first without weights and then with – noticing how you react to the addition of resistance.

Here's how this approach would work with the squat, an exercise which provides a wonderful opportunity to 'work on yourself' in addition to toning the glutes and hamstrings. We will study it further in Chapter 7, with the addition of weights.

The question that concerns us here is: how do we start the squat? The key is not to initiate the movement by shortening or pulling down. So often, squatting begins with the neck

tightening and the head pulled back and down into the spine. This serves to compress the spine, placing additional and unnecessary stress on this area. In fact, you don't have to 'do' anything to go down – gravity provides all the help you need. Instead, what matters is 'undoing', or letting go.

If you recall the Alexander Technique procedure called 'Monkey', the pupil is instructed to 'think up' in order to maintain length and to initiate the bend by releasing the ankles. This allows the knees to go forward and away, which in turn causes the body to lose height – but not length. In other words, at no time is bending (which should be performed with the ankle, knee and hip joints) allowed to cause shortening in the torso. Success in performing the squat will depend on inhibiting the automatic response to 'go down' when squatting – that is, thinking that bending the knees requires us to shorten the spine.

Preventing the wrong things from happening right from the start is the key to performing any exercise successfully. In the case of the squat, it is the necessity to think 'up' in order to go down. This requires us to ensure that the heels are in contact with the floor so that we have something to think 'up' from. Also, that the movement is initiated in the correct sequence, beginning with the ankles, the knees and then the hips. Starting the bend with the hips, without freeing the ankles, risks pushing the hips forwards and hollowing the lower back, which creates unnecessary strain in that area.

CASE STUDY
Fitness at work

'The challenge was not to respond to my habit of competitive end-gaining.'

I have always been interested in sport and exercise. I have a natural love of movement and hate sitting at a desk looking at a screen, something I did for more than ten years. That is why I decided to take part-time work that was more physically demanding. I started a gruelling job lifting boxes most of the day. This was my chance to get active and be paid for it.

I found that others had come to the job with the same intention as me, but it became evident that they were tired and stiff at the end of the day with no increase in their fitness. Being an Alexander Technique teacher, I thought that this would not apply to me. Well, I was in for a surprise!

At the end of the day I was also feeling tired and tight. On arriving home I would shower, spend half an hour lying in semi-supine, legs up against the wall, then stretch. The stretching in particular gave me much relief from the tightness in my muscles. But how could I move in a way that would prevent this tightening? Maybe it wasn't such a good idea to have taken this job after all. What happened to the smooth, blissful movement I had learned through the Alexander Technique?

Resisting the temptation to resign, I decided to make it a challenge to prove that the Technique works in all environments. At first, I spent a lot of time observing others and I was not surprised that they felt tired and tight at the end of the day. I noticed that they moved in a 'narrowing' way, not allowing freedom in their hips and at the top of their spine. Most bent in the classic, end-gaining manner – from the thoracic spine rather than at the hips. Was I also doing this but unaware of it? Surely, I reasoned, we can move in an expansive, non-end-gaining way at work, which enables the appropriate muscles to stretch as well as contract?

The workplace was very busy, with incentives to reach targets, which reduced my self-awareness. So my first move was to ensure that I spent my lunch break lying in semi-supine to help bring back some awareness. Fortunately, the company had created a quiet room where there was a couch. I gave myself an extra 30 minutes for my lunch break so I could have this expansive time. I found this very useful, bringing back some level of awareness of myself and so enabling my directions to allow more freedom and balance.

I noticed that most of my end-gaining habits were derived from peer pressure. Later, I concluded that I imposed this on myself. This pressure played on my fears, such as thinking I was not strong enough and I had to be quicker. Recognize this tendency in the gym? So I asked myself: what would happen if I did not respond to my fear? I decided that I would give myself more time to find my own internal rhythm and move from my centre of gravity.

From this way of thinking, my integrated self emerged – with my spine supporting me and my weight falling through my feet. As I started to move and interact in this way, I discovered that I did not need to stretch as much at the end of the day, a sign that I was moving more expansively. My stamina increased, as well as my flexibility. I began to notice more grounded movement from flexible ankle joints. My head was balancing freely on top of my spine instead of being fixed and pushed back. I stopped accommodating my movement from my projected belief about someone else's judgements of me. I recognized that the quality of my movement depended on the quality of my thoughts.

Some days I would be slower and weaker. The challenge was not to respond to my habit of competitive end-gaining but to 'inhibit'. Other days I would get really stuck and feel fed-up. I would then ask myself how I could build a presence about me to kick-start true inhibition. Making the steps or goals smaller was the key to initiating this process and reminding myself of what I wanted: namely, the freedom to move expansively.

Alison Broome

CASE STUDY
Martial arts

'Instead of hunching up to fight, I stretched out.'

I developed an interest in martial arts during my late teens and early 20s, when I began serious training. I had always been an active sportsman, playing rugby and racket sports, but I gradually replaced the rugby training with martial arts. I was fascinated by the precision and grace of Chinese kung fu, not to mention the power and confidence it offered.

The training was tough, seeking to develop the cardiovascular fitness, speed and strength necessary for fighting. Indeed, the term 'fighting fit' is very apt. At the time I was built like Popeye, with lots of muscles. I'm sure my constitution has what bodybuilders term 'flair' – namely, the ability to gain lean muscle mass very easily. If I got hit, this usually caused my opponent as much pain as it did me.

My first experience of the Alexander Technique came quite by chance. I was working on a farm, the owner of which had been known as the 'wheelchair farmer' because he had spent a long time in a chair with an unresolved back problem. That is, until he began taking Alexander lessons. A teacher would sometimes arrive at the farm to teach the family and, when I asked her about the Technique, she said that she couldn't tell me but could demonstrate it. So I had a trial lesson, which was a turning point in my life. More followed. I remember her laughing when, after a few lessons, I reported the steady disappearance of symptoms and wondered if this was anything to do with what she was teaching me!

When I applied the idea of 'forward and up' to running, the results were astounding. I knocked eight minutes off my usual time for 4.8km (3 miles). Instead of concentrating on the running itself, my attention was on the idea of lengthening the spine and releasing the head from the top. The run was effortless! I resolved to use this approach in all my other training, producing real improvements in stamina, balance and flexibility.

Instead of hunching up to fight, I stretched out. The experience was of having more time to think and react in response to my opponent, although shrinking under attack was still the automatic option. The style and precision of my forms also improved, as did my balance while executing difficult moves. A key difference was that I knew where my body was in much more detail. I found I could stop the form, analyse my intention for movement and recognize, then correct, erroneous ideas. Before, the habits were triggered before they could be modified, so the same old faults would happen time and again.

I finally gained a place on an Alexander Technique teacher-training course. The intensity of this work led me to question the physical training regimes I practised for kung fu, particularly the speed at which they were performed. Some of this, I'm sure, was to encourage quickness of reaction, but I was more dissatisfied with an ongoing lack of consciousness. I was not able to attend to the coordination of the whole while training under duress and so began to work on my own routines, where I could control the speed and apply more thought to the integration of the whole rather than specific muscle groups.

Near the end of my Alexander training I took up tai chi, and this presented the perfect opportunity to combine the quality of consciousness I was developing in the Alexander Technique with a martial art. I did less and less physical training yet found no loss of ability when sparring with my kung fu colleagues.

The Alexander Technique has allowed me to be much more discerning in all my physical training, enabling me to develop aspects which enhance ability and drop those which are superfluous or even interfere with my development. The result is greater power of choice, and a sense of self which I never had before.

David Bainbridge

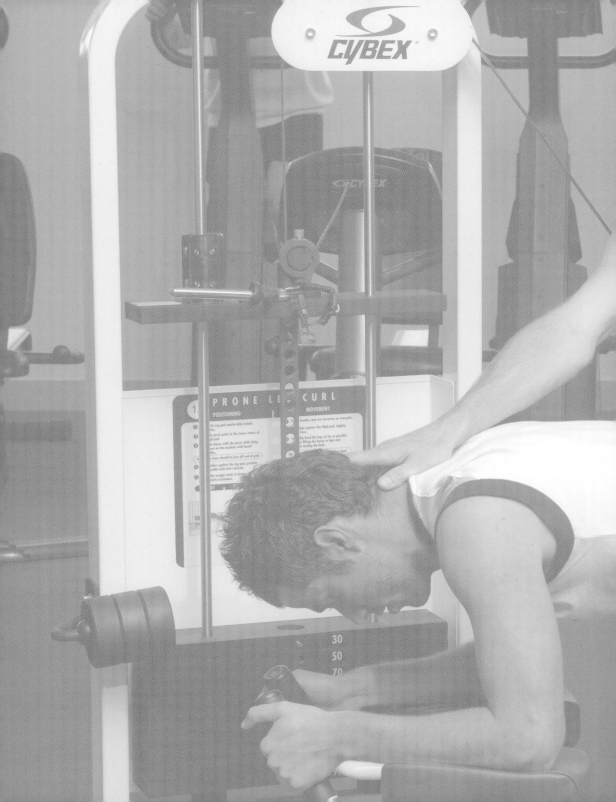

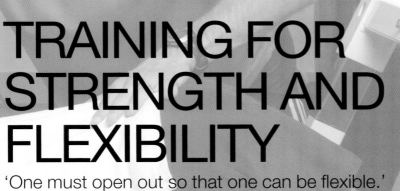

7

TRAINING FOR STRENGTH AND FLEXIBILITY

'One must open out so that one can be flexible.'

Merce Cunningham

Most golf and tennis magazines promote an illusion. Namely, that you can learn to do anything from a book. It's like thinking you can tell what cherry cola tastes like from someone describing it to you. The 'real thing' is not how we imagine it to be. Anyone who has ever tried to learn how to strike a golf ball by following an instruction manual on the subject (often penned by the greats of the sport) and has then gone out and attempted to 'hit like Tiger' will recognize this fallacy, probably from bitter experience.

Rather than reacting to inevitable disappointment with the infantile frustration of a two-year-old who can't have everything he wants right now, treat the experience for what it's worth: as a stimulus for considered response to an activity that demands considerable sensory input as well as verbal and written cues.

We should all include resistance training in our workout schedule. As the saying goes, 'There's nothing wrong with being strong.' We begin losing muscle mass in our mid-30s, to the point that at the age of about 70 we've lost half of what we once had. If we don't do anything about it, that is. In contrast, even people in the eighth decade of life have shown major gains in useable strength by following a simple programme of resistance training.

John Jerome puts this beautifully, in his book On Turning 65: 'One distressing thing that is slipping away as we age is our comfort zone: the part of the physical world that we operate unthinkingly with ease and grace and efficiency. That sphere of activity begins to shrink as surely

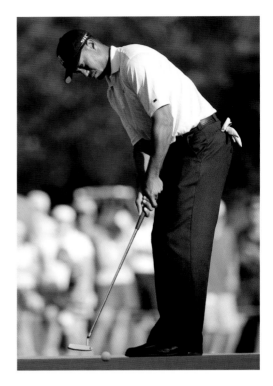

Above Even the best do not rest on their laurels. In addition to driving, chipping and putting, Tiger Woods apparently spends time every day working on his balance.

as our connective tissue. That's what we oldsters must train for: usefulness; the ability to bring muscle to bear. The problem isn't that you no longer have anything to bring, it's that you can't find it to bring it. You can't recruit it. You have to practise recruitment. In fact, that's specifically how practice works: without it you forget where those motor units are. You forget their location, their very address in the computer sense of the term. Motor units… are accessible to the will. They are how the mind finds the muscle. Muscle is function. The motor unit, the unit of muscular effort, gives you a way of putting your shoulder directly to the wheel of age – if not to roll it back, then at least to slow its progress.'

One of the major issues affecting our response to the weights room is that, particularly for men, it involves the big head as well as the little one. Just as we blithely believe we can read a couple of chapters on how to execute a topspin backhand then head off to our local courts and play like Roger Federer, so our approach to resistance training is complicated by macho attitudes, preconceptions and a large amount of assumed knowledge. However, if we are truly to master the art of working out, we need to foster a state of mind that makes weight training safe, interesting, productive and useable by thinking into the activity.

Free weights or machines?

Free weights have disappeared from many gyms in the belief that they are more difficult to master and pose a greater risk of injury than machine-based resistance systems. In addition, they have a strongly masculine image that can be off-putting to novices and women.

This is a pity, since free weights offer multi-dimensional, neuromuscular and musculo-skeletal training that is superior to that provided by machines. The latter tend to have fixed planes of movement and user positions, such as sitting and lying, that minimize the training effect on the body's major stabilizing muscles. Free weights offer the chance to move in any direction in space, without restriction – and to

develop our kinaesthetic awareness and good use while we do so.

Whichever method you prefer, your approach should first be to acknowledge that the weight is the stimulus which is trying to put you wrong. Take time to observe someone working on a machine or with free weights to get an idea of how the particular exercise might affect your use. Not only will this forewarn you as to the potential dangers, there is something about watching another gymster doing something badly that will warm the cockles of

Below Weight is the stimulus that is trying to put you wrong. It's vital, therefore, to attend to one's general use before going into movement.

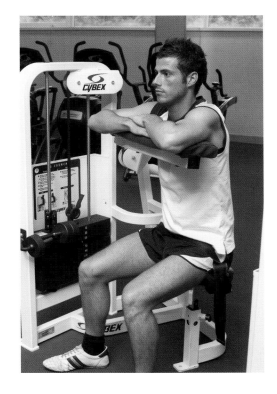

your heart – so don't deprive yourself of this sordid pleasure! Armed with an idea of both what to do and what to avoid, you are ready to start taking some calculated risks.

Biceps curl

The curl (along with the pec-deck) is an exercise that raises the question of muscular over-development. Some guys seem determined to use it to build Popeye arms (just as they are eager to sprout pecs you could rest a glass of water on while standing up). However, what seems at first to be a straightforward, 'do it in your sleep' kind of routine – bending the elbows while holding a weighted bar or dumb-bells – has, in fact, different phases which increase the potential for misuse. The upward phase, when the hands move closer to the upper arm, is the concentric phase in which the muscles shorten following a contraction against the resistance they are overcoming. The downward phase is the eccentric phase, when the muscles lengthen as external forces overcome them.

That's the theory. In practice, though, whenever our hands get busy, be it holding a weight or typing on a keyboard or moving heavy objects, other parts of our body want to join the party. First it's the shoulders creeping forwards and up towards the ears, then the neck has to put in its two cents' worth, which means the head becomes pulled down. As the muscles fatigue, so the knees lock, the buttocks clench, the lower back arches and the hips thrust forward in a bid to complete the tough concentric phase. What starts as a simple desire for well-defined upper arms can quickly deteriorate into a maelstrom of muscular misuse. Watch most people tackling a set of curls and, assuming the weight they are using is heavy enough to pose a challenge, you will see a demonstration of most of these unwanted and potentially damaging elements.

This is not a criticism of curls per se. Anyone who has tried lifting a sleeping four-year-old out of a car seat at midnight will know that strong arms are an asset. However, executing effective curls does not mean contracting your body into a parody of Rodin's *The Thinker*.

Rather than thinking of muscles shortening when they contract, think of them gliding – as in the teeth of two combs sliding over each other as they are pushed together. To compare the difference, first tense the biceps in your right arm, then bend the elbow upward a few times. Next, with your left elbow, don't tense anything but simply bend the elbow while imagining the biceps fibres gliding over each another.

Now think about the effect that the movement is having on the relationship between your head, neck and spine. See if you can perform the curl with absolutely no sign of strain, no indication that you're lifting a big weight – and at the same time sing your national anthem in a voice that doesn't sound like you're giving birth. You will probably find your muscles fatiguing more quickly – in which case, cut the number of repetitions, reduce the weight you are lifting and treat any mocking comments from your fellow gym-users with the disdain they deserve.

Squat

This exercise is often accompanied by a warning that it can damage knees, back or both. However, our response should be to note that one of the biggest contributors to the modern plague known as lower back pain is sitting on the sofa, and that we need not be afraid of this potentially terrific exercise.

Unlike many other parts of the world, squatting is not a feature of Western society. This is a pity. It is a skill that helps us to develop good balance, coordination and use. With a loaded bar across the shoulders, it also builds muscular strength and endurance.

When you watch this exercise performed in most gyms, however, you can see why it has a bad reputation. With lower back arched, head crunched so far back it practically touches the shoulders and eyes fixed on the ceiling in a heavenly plea, it's the gesture of a wannabe saint rather than an intelligent exerciser.

First, attempt to squat without any additional weight. Free your neck, lengthen your torso while retaining the spine's natural curvature, release your knees out over your toes and keep your heels on the ground. Only when you can do this satisfactorily should you add weight.

Some people think that putting a weight on their shoulders is a great excuse to tighten everything up, starting with their neck. It should be just the opposite. Nor should doing this cause you to shorten your back. In fact, done properly, the squat will help your back do what it's meant to do ordinarily – namely, lengthen and resist against the force of gravity.

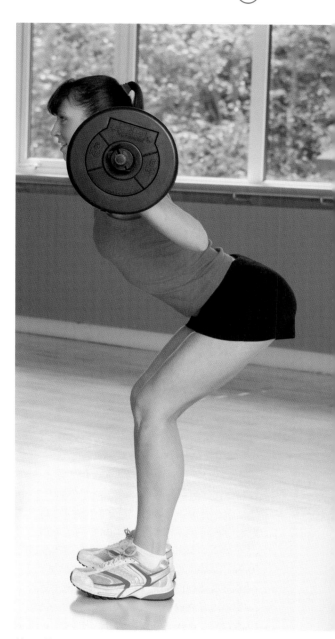

Above This approach to squatting is often seen in the gym and bears little resemblance to the natural squat shown on p.111 or the powerful squat used by the Olympic lifter on p.81. It loads the lower back excessively.

One of the key moments in squatting is when you begin the upward phase of the movement. Looking up towards the ceiling or even a wall mirror in front of you is not going to help. In fact, it is going to add unnecessary compressive forces to your already loaded spine. Therefore, do not initiate the upward movement with an increase in neck tension. You need to put your thought where it's really going to help: your feet and your back. Think of sending your heels down (to avoid overloading the knees) and lifting your back up. This will avoid loading any one part of the spine and will carry you smoothly back to your starting point. Done correctly, squats will give you the power and confidence to carry that heavy box up three flights of stairs, which your husband didn't have time for because he had to get to his workout!

For an interesting variation, we have Dan Barach, Alexander Technique teacher and musician, to thank. According to Barach, Chinese legend has it that one hundred wall squats each day will cure anything! So what's a wall squat? Face a wall with your feet as close to each other and to the wall as you can manage without losing your balance. If you need a little elevation, place a telephone directory under your heels (and, as you become more confident, regularly tear out a handful of pages). As you squat, the wall in front of you serves as a reminder to maintain length in the back while minimising your forward lean. It also serves as a reference for how vertically we descend. Sometimes there is a tendency to pull to one side or the other.

Dead lift

Place weight on bar, bend and lift to a standing position. Repeat X number of times. Simple?

The dead lift is a great exercise because it is transferable to everyday life, such as when we need to shift a bag of cement, paving slabs or a case of wine without herniating ourselves. However, the problem with the move, as many doctors will attest, is that if carried out incorrectly, it can place considerable strain on your back. Like the squat, it often receives a bad press.

First of all, we need inhibition and direction in order to get down to a level to grasp the bar. Before bending, pause and give your directions for squatting: release the front of the ankles and the back of the knees, with the knees releasing forward and away while maintaining the length and natural curves of the spine and freedom in the neck. This is not the same as the traditional admonition to 'Keep your back straight', and causes much less loading – that is, unnecessary strain – on the knees and lower back. It's also stronger: the resistance of a curved column is directly proportional to the square of its number of curvatures plus one, so that a naturally curved spine offers ten times the resistance to loading compared to a straight column of the same dimensions.

The lift itself is basically the reverse of what you did to grasp the bar in the first place – except, of course, that you have the resistance

Right Working on the dead lift: the back is lengthening, tension in the neck is reduced to appropriate levels, and power comes from the connection into the floor, through the hips and into a balanced head-neck-back relationship.

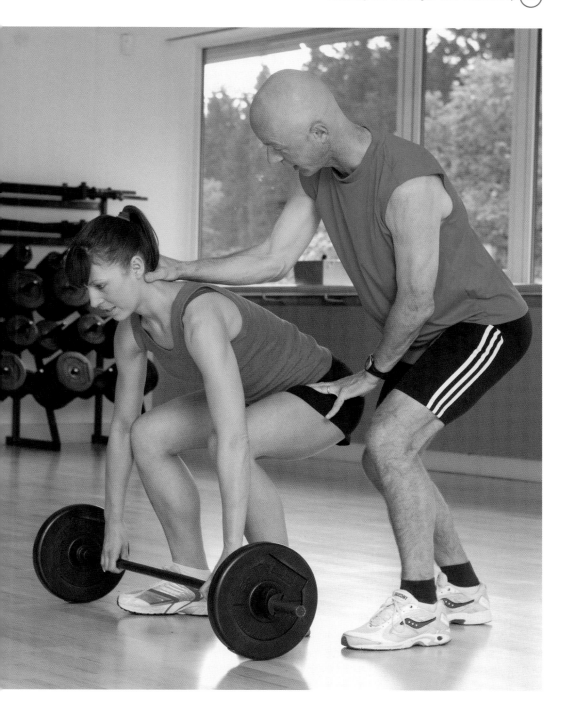

provided by the bar to deal with. Again, inhibition and direction provide a solution.

There is sometimes a tendency to overreact to weight, and in response to overload certain parts of the body, particularly the lower back. The load needs to be distributed throughout the body, and jerking or overreacting can do just the opposite. In the learning stages it's therefore important to work slowly and carefully. If you use a sufficiently light weight, it will serve as a stimulus to (a) tell you when you are lifting incorrectly and (b) help you develop greater strength and coordination. As your practical intelligence grows with experience, you can begin to add more weight.

Between sets – you know, the time when you're usually admiring either yourself or someone else in the mirror, or are slumped on a bench 'recovering' – go into 'Monkey' (see Chapter 5). Lightly holding a bar, pole or bench to maintain balance and achieve a slightly more vertical position than you might otherwise be able to, practise moving in and out of a deep squat. See how free, smooth, connected and effortless you can make this.

Use the mirror to see if your body is as vertical as you believe it to be – you may be in for a surprise. This kind of recovery will help you develop better technique when you next lift, with your awareness, energy and coordination greatly enhanced.

Pec-deck

Whatever your opinion on the merits of this particular piece of equipment, we take the view that no exercise or machine is intrinsically evil.

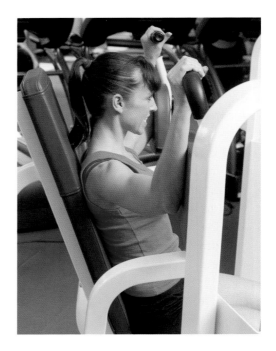

Above The pec-deck is a machine on which we must react actively by maintaining a sense of lengthening and connection through the sitting bones and feet, and being aware of the tendency for the back to arch.

Arguments can be made regarding the functionality of the exercise or its relevance to your sense of balance, but you might choose to do it because you like pumped-up pectorals. So be it.

In a seated position, the arms are raised, bent at the elbow and placed behind two padded bars which are connected to a resistance. The idea is to bring your arms together in front of you, working against the resistance in an effort to build a bigger and sexier chest.

Following the suggestion to observe someone using the machine to get an idea of what you might want to anticipate and avoid, look for several tendencies:

As the arms open to their extreme 'don't shoot' position, they tend to hyperextend behind the shoulders because of the pull of the resistance. This results in the back arching, the pelvis tilting and bodyweight being dropped on to the thighs instead of remaining in the sitting bones. There's also a tendency to pull the head back against the rest, thus flattening the natural curve in the neck. With feet resting passively on the foot rest, the legs are disengaged.

In order to overcome the resistance and begin the movement to bring the arms together in front of the body (the concentric phase, otherwise known as 'the hard bit'), most people continue to arch their spine and pull their head back. This creates a great deal of unnecessary and unwanted tension in the neck and shoulders as well as excessive pressure on the lower (thoracic) spine. This will undoubtedly affect the person's breathing, as arching the back fixes the lower ribs and makes it impossible to allow free movement in this area. Lack of engagement and direction in the legs, and the lack of any link into the feet, means balancing on two points – the thighs – rather than on four. This makes it much more difficult to maintain the integrity (length and width) of the back.

Forearmed is forewarned: now at least we know what to expect if we just go at this exercise blindly, trusting our innate talent and overall athleticism to guide us. Instead, we decide to proceed with caution, starting with a reasonably light weight and paying attention to

our use as we get the feel of the machine. It's important to notice how the machine tends to 'sculpt' us, to encourage or even provoke us into assuming positions that mitigate against good use.

If, however, we do not react passively to what the machine wants us to do but instead react actively by consciously maintaining a sense of lengthening and connection through the main points of support – namely the sitting bones and feet – we exploit the machine to strengthen our sense of good use. So we don't allow the machine to cause us to arch our back, we don't pull our head back against the pad, we check to see that the weight is going down through our sitting bones, we aim the knees out over the toes and we send a strong message to our heels to release into the ground. And when we initiate the movement, it's not with a tightening of the neck, but by employing the natural give and elasticity at the end of the eccentric phase of the exercise.

Seated leg extension

This machine is designed to build up the quadriceps, the big muscle group at the front of the thigh. From a seated position, the ankles are tucked behind a padded bar, which is then raised as the legs are straightened. At the end of the concentric phase we are sitting with our legs straight out in front of us.

As soon as the effort needed to raise the bar passes one's comfort zone, the exercise can degenerate into a morass of misuse. In trying to work the quadriceps harder, we risk generating unwarranted tension throughout our

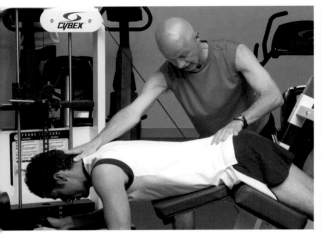
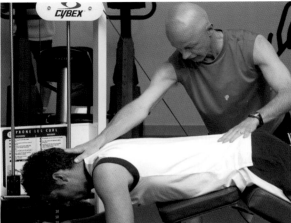

Above, left and right A key to the effective use of resistance machines is to not react passively to what the machine wants us to do. Here, in the leg curl, it's possible to exploit the machine to strengthen the sense of good use.

system. The powerful urge to tighten the neck and pull down in front, while losing the connection of the sitting bones on the seat, can completely overwhelm our initial desire to do otherwise. In terms of the cost/benefit ratio, performing with the normal 'more has got to be better' mentality, the gains in quad strength will be overshadowed by the unnecessary effort you are generating everywhere else. What an opportunity for change and growth!

As is so often the case, a seemingly easy exercise can provide a wealth of material for the thinking gymster. After all, end-gaining is only an extra weight away. 'Going for it' can unconsciously become your normal gym mode: get on the machine, grind out the set and move on.

While there is a certain amount of pleasure to be gained from achieving your targets on a

given day, bringing an awareness of good use into the equation will make the process that much more satisfying and, in the end, more beneficial.

Press-ups

It's a myth that being able to perform press-ups is a function of pure arm strength – which is one reason why women in particular tend not to attempt this excellent upper-body exercise or stick to modified versions of it. Instead, we can take a more skilful approach to the press-up in which the emphasis is not on how much the arms have to work, but how little.

First we need to establish our primary pattern – the orientation of our head, neck and back. This is directly related to our standing pattern: poor standing posture will follow, like a bad lunch, into the press-up. Dropping the hips creates an exaggerated arch in the lower back, which compromises the integrity of the spine as well as restricting movement of the lower ribs. This in turn limits breathing (try arching your back and taking a deep breath at the same time). The neck will tend to shorten if the shoulders become overly involved, with the head dropping on descent and pulling back on ascent, creating unnecessary strain in the neck, shoulders and upper back.

However, if the head leads and the body follows (with the back lengthening and widening), the whole body maintains its integrity despite the demands of being in a horizontal rather than vertical position. The 'right' condition of the primary pattern is established and reinforced at the beginning of the movement, rather than after the movement has already begun. It is much more difficult to try and change a movement after the 'wrong' conditions have set in.

We need to maintain integrity without compromising the ability of our lower ribs to expand freely and easily during the movement. In other words, we don't stiffen the body to maintain a correct position, we energize it to maintain the right orientation without fixing the ribs. This is not the same as forced inhalation and exhalation, but the natural response of the breath to the demands and rhythm of the movement.

The head should lead the spine into length and not drop (taking the neck with it) in a misguided attempt to shorten the downward section of the exercise. In other words, although the movement in space is vertical, the internal movement along the spine is horizontal. The shoulders are not overly solicited and the shoulder blades are not raised. As our bodyweight drops, we rebound off our hands

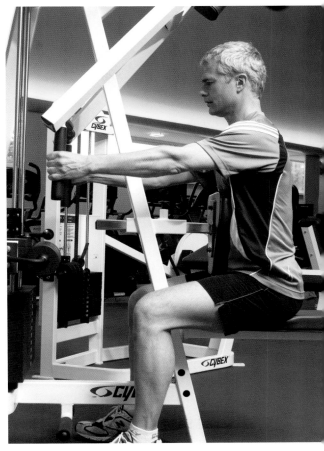

Above Too many exercisers jump on a resistance machine without adjusting any of the settings. Even a seemingly simple exercise such as a seated row can provide a wealth of material for the thinking gymster.

on the way back up.

At the start of each repetition, pause to re-establish the integrity of the primary movement; to release any unnecessary tension; to free up any holding; to renew orientation; and to re-energize the whole self. In this way, the humble press-up becomes an expression of vigour and vitality rather than a feat of strength.

'Cheating'

'Cheating' doesn't have to involve performance-enhancing drugs. It also refers to the use of ballistic action (such as bouncing or swinging) or some other means to complete a movement in strength training that could not be achieved using strict form or conventional 'good technique'. For example, rather than letting the biceps do all the work to complete a curl, the 'cheater' might throw his hips forward and lean backward to get the bar past the 'sticking point' at which the movement becomes most difficult.

Proponents of the 'strict form' school of strength training argue that cheating is bad (as the name implies) because poor form increases the risk of injury as well as diverting effort to unwanted areas – in the case of the curl, from biceps to shoulders. The 'cheater' is also accused of being able to achieve a result by unfair advantage – by swinging the bar and thus avoiding the work necessary to get a 'real' result. From an Alexander perspective, this can be interpreted and condemned as a classic form of end-gaining: achieve the goal regardless of the cost.

Hold on there! Cheating is actually what we do naturally, in everyday life, to move large objects efficiently. Anyone who has needed to lug a heavy suitcase into the boot of a car will appreciate the contribution that momentum makes to the process. Swinging the damn thing up on to the edge of the bumper, then sliding it in the rest of the way is a lot easier than trying to hoist it in following strict lifting protocols.

Another danger of being too strict is that exercise becomes 'unnatural', in the sense that it no longer mimics the kinds of movement found in 'the real world'. For example, when we lift (i.e. curl) a child up in our arms, we don't hold our elbows tight to our sides and keep our back perfectly straight. Nor do we worry too much if our legs help a little in getting the toddler over the 'sticking point'. When we try too hard to maintain a high standard of strictness, there is a risk that our bodies become rigid and 'held' in an effort to prevent unwanted movement. If good technique encourages rigidity and holding, what does bad technique do?

So what's the bottom line? Unconscious cheating is risky, while being overly strict can lead to a style of movement that is robotic and lacks flow. Finding a balance and making considered choices is easier when we combine a knowledge of good technique with a sense of good use.

Flexibility

Stretching is a bit like flossing our teeth. We don't do it as much as we should. As a result, muscles, ligaments and tendons that once allowed us to touch our toes easily become tighter if we don't work to keep them long. Sometimes, even everyday movements can become difficult as our bodies literally seize up.

How often do we finish a workout and head straight for the shower (or the bar), without

Right Two examples of stretching ability. Natural facility can make good use easier, but it doesn't necessarily make it a conscious choice. We can all practise 'thinking in activity'.

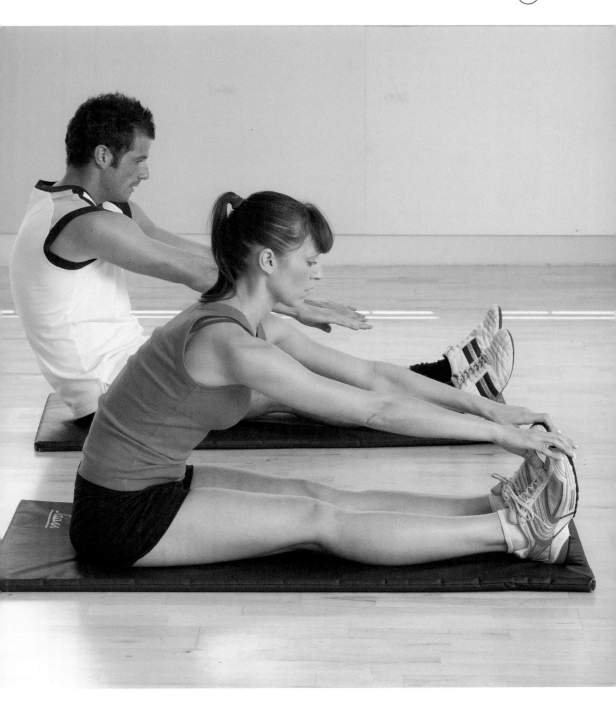

taking advantage of the warmth in our bodies to maintain and extend the range of movement in our joints and muscles? Regular stretching can also have a positive impact on posture while offering a great opportunity to cultivate good use.

However, stretching can often seem like hard work for little benefit. Surely the strain of trying to get your fingers to reach your toes far outweighs the possible gains in the length of your hamstring? If you tighten six muscles in order to stretch three, is it worth it?

How, then, do we evaluate our approach to flexibility training? In his book The Alexander Technique As I See It, Patrick Macdonald gives us a different and potentially revolutionary criterion with which we can judge:

'It is possible to demonstrate two forces, or sets of forces, acting in the human body and, in particular, along the spine. These forces may possibly have something in common with the positive and negative of Western science, or the Chinese yin and yang. "Force A" has a tendency to contract and distort. It is closely allied to the pull of gravity and causes a heaviness in the body, which is not the heaviness of avoirdupois. "Force B" has an expansionary or elongatory tendency. It is often referred to, in a general way, as "life". It produces lightness in the body. I take it to be the natural, though not any longer the normal, condition.'

When we stretch, it is useful to know whether in doing so we are reinforcing Force A or Force B. Could we learn to prevent the former and encourage the latter? Alexander, you may recall, found that his kinaesthetic sense

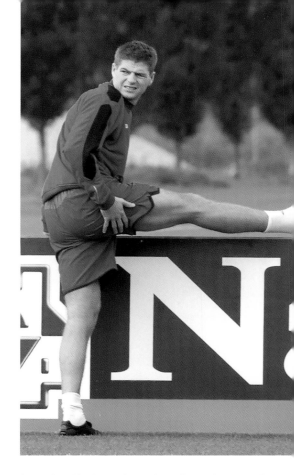

Above Stretching is too often performed in a perfunctory and half-hearted manner, as shown here by England footballer Steven Gerrard – whose attention is clearly not focused on his hamstrings.

was not always accurate, in that he often felt he was doing things correctly when in fact he wasn't. Learning to recognize this is one of the most important and most challenging aspects of good stretching. One can assume the right position, avoid straining and breathe into the stretch yet still be letting Force A dominate – and not be aware that this is happening.

In his book *Staying Supple*, John Jerome offers other criteria:

- Don't hurt yourself!
- Stretch what feels good, for as long as it feels good to do so.
- Pay attention.
- Be patient, for it takes time to develop and maintain suppleness.

Of crucial importance, then, is our attitude. Call it 'beginner's mind'. How we go about stretching will strongly affect both the process and the results. How often have we found ourselves wallowing in self-congratulatory bliss during a stretching session, only to be pulled up short when reality, in the form of a glance in the mirror, suggests much more attention is needed to the downward pull being generated in the spine?

Standard doctrine says that in passive stretching you should hold the stretch for around 30 seconds. Jerome, in contrast, suggests: 'You want to hold each stretch just as long as it holds your attention – when your mind begins to wander, stretch something else.' Because stretching can easily become routine, mechanical and boring, we often look for something more interesting to help pass the time. However, noticing if we are present or not brings us back to the moment. Expanding your awareness to include the bit(s) being stretched and its effect on your head-neck-back relationship adds an important dimension to the process.

We can all can sit on a gym mat, lean forward, grab a foot and execute a hamstring stretch. And there is, of course, a certain sense of accomplishment as the hamstring releases

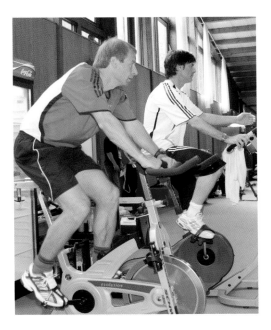

Above Even great sports players like the German international footballer and national team coach Jurgen Klinsmann need to pay attention while exercising. The seat of his bike is placed too far back, forcing his weight forward and contracting his neck. The person on his left has a more efficient set-up.

and it's possible to hold more and more of the foot. However, it gets much more interesting when you direct the head-neck-back relationship at the same time.

First of all, you will not be in such a rush to grab more foot (a common indicator of 'successful' hamstring stretching). Take a little time to 'think up' and you will find that this is already bringing gentle tension into the hamstring.

Now lean forward while working to maintain a sense of length. Notice your breathing, often overlooked as you move into position, and let it tell you how far and how fast to extend the movement. As soon as you lose interest in the hamstring being stretched, switch legs and repeat the process.

By now you will be more aware both of the stretch itself and how it's connecting to and affecting the rest of your self. You might pay attention to the resistance in your lower back, inhibiting any urge to pull right through it in order to grab more of your foot.

This is very different from the typical mechanical, 'get it over' approach. It leaves you feeling less rushed, less impatient, and less liable to become frustrated at any perceived lack of progress.

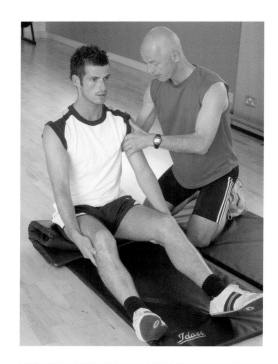

Stretching the Alexander way

- Take time to decide what you are stretching, why and how. There are many different approaches, each with its own rationale and list of claimed benefits. These range from the classic 'stretch and hold for 30 seconds' technique, to moving a limb repetitively through an increasing range of movement, to stretching and actively resisting the stretch at the same time, to assisted stretching where a partner takes you further than you could go yourself. Finding the approach that most interests and works for you is a matter of personal preference.

- Learn the correct action needed to perform the stretch, including an understanding of what to do and also what to avoid. It is vital that you identify and eliminate potentially damaging practices. In other words, use

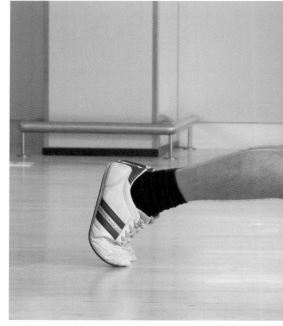

Left Failure to make a choice is a form of misuse. Better choices (back lengthening, legs released, a folded mat beneath the buttocks) produce a less contorted and more effective hamstring stretch.

yourself well while you stretch. If you have comparatively short hamstring tendons, what is the point of bending in the middle of your back and straining with your neck and shoulders just to reach your foot?

● Inhibit your urge to jump right into the stretch. Say to yourself: 'I have…time.' Time to prevent tightening or muscling into the stretch.

● Don't leave your brain in the changing room. In other words, stretch actively, pay attention and be interested in the process as well as the result.

● Like any other gym activity, stretching is a skill which will improve and develop according to your attitude towards it.

Core stability

No fitness centre today is complete without a core training programme, and gym balls and balance boards have become part of the furniture. Core training focuses on the deep trunk muscles, founded on the belief that strengthening these specific areas will stabilize

Below In core stability work, maintaining the integrity of primary control sets the correct overall tone of the exercise. Here, the demands of the exercise overwhelm the exerciser's ability to maintain a good head-neck-back relationship.

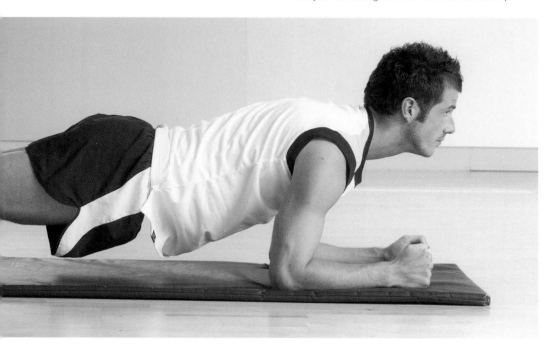

the spine, thus reducing injuries and improving performance. Judging from the general state of collapse in which most people exist these days, there is clearly a need for this type of exercise. Like cholesterol, though, there's good and bad core training.

Since few children suffer from lower back pain, we can assume that core stability is something we lose along the way, like baby teeth. There is the famous story of a top decathlete who tried to imitate a child's activities and had to retire exhausted after an hour spent copying the youngster's naturally free and undistorted movement. I'm sure some personal trainers would say our decathlete probably needed to spend more time on the gym ball, but it's fair to assume that the youngster didn't do any specific fitness training at all and still outlasted his eminent elder.

Most approaches to core training aim directly at the weakness and try to strengthen muscles which have weakened over the years. However, many generally prescribed exercises can place high levels of stress on the lower

Below This yoga position, known as upward-facing dog, is a great illustration of how to stretch the front of the torso without unduly contracting the neck and pulling the head into the spine.

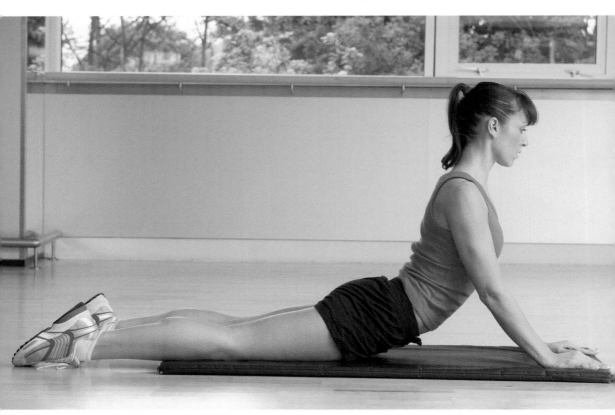

back. For example, in 'Superman' (performed by lying flat on the stomach and raising the upper body and legs off the floor), the lumbar spine pays a very high compression penalty, which transfers load to the facet joints and crushes the interspinous ligaments. Better, instead, is to address the causes of that weakness by recognizing patterns of misuse and faulty sensory awareness.

A crucial aim of the Alexander Technique is to inform every part of the body with thought.

Below Same exercise, completely different outcome. Note the sharply retracted head, which makes the lack of flexibility through the lower spine and torso more apparent.

Learning how to direct your energy in activity is the key to good functioning. Let's say you've been given the oft-prescribed advice in core classes to pull your belly button towards your spine. Carrying out this advice with too much enthusiasm will contract the rectus abdominus and pull you down. What's more, if you already slouch (pull down) as a response to gravity, strengthening your core will only make matters worse.

This will further increase the distorting and contractive influence of gravity (what the Alexander Technique teacher Patrick Macdonald called 'Force A' energy),

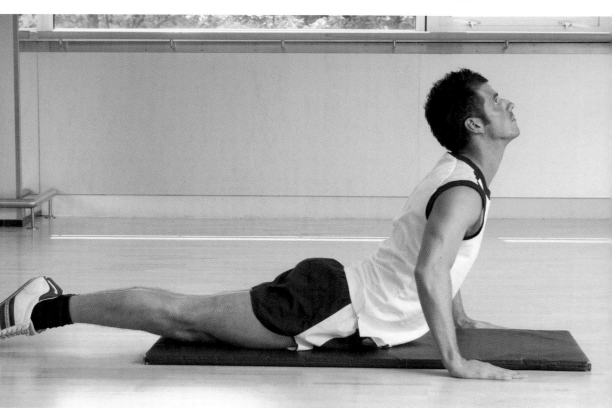

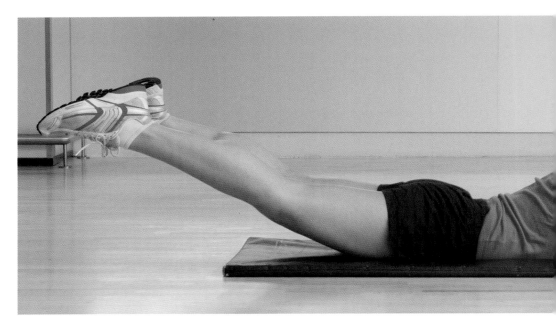

compressing the spine as well as interfering with breathing. Not good! Engaging the lower abdominal muscles while maintaining a strong sense of lengthening is a more balanced response.

Since many people today suffer from poor posture, we can assume that their anti-gravity response is weak as well. They're lacking in what Macdonald called 'Force B' energy. Learning to generate more Force B – lengthening and lightening in response to the downward pressure of gravity – can greatly improve the organization of the lower back.

Discover how much Force B you can generate by sitting at the edge of a chair with your back unsupported, maintaining a free and lengthened head, neck and spine, and see how long you last before fatiguing and reverting to a more familiar slump. The child in our earlier

example would be able to remain balanced in this position almost indefinitely. What allows children to do this with such apparent ease is not a well defined six-pack or rippling back extensors, but inherently good primary control of use producing a natural, undistorted quality of movement.

Putting bigger shock absorbers and go-faster stripes on your car won't transform you into the next Michael Schumacher. Poor driving habits will follow you into a Ferrari as easily as a Ford. Bending, sitting, picking things up and putting on shoes all require a certain amount of skill and awareness to be done effectively. It is very easy just to 'do' them and move on.

One may assume that after a session spent strengthening one's core, there is no longer any need for attention and skill. Big mistake. Casual observation of teachers and participants

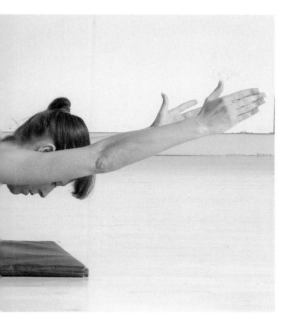

relaxing after a strenuous gym ball workout seemed to indicate that the awareness encouraged during the class was left behind in the studio. Watching them slump cross-legged over a revitalizing drink, the impression was that they were more than happy to give their aching cores a rest and revert to an unthinking posture. It's vital that we recognize the need for a link between thought and action – and that at all times we train our brains while we train our muscles.

Left In 'Superman', strength and flexibility combine in a wonderful attitude of grace and flow.

Below The way we go about training strongly affects both the process and the results. It's important to take time to prepare both body and mind for an exercise.

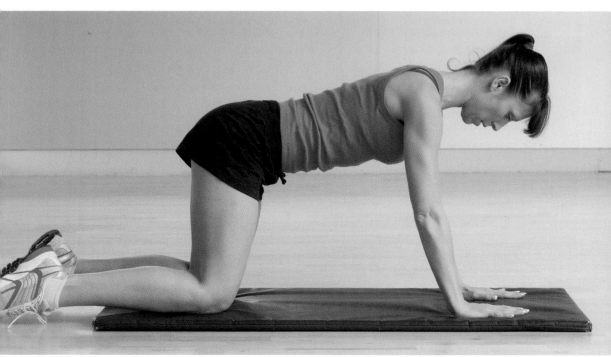

Resistance training and powerlifting

'What Alexander Technique brings to resistance training is subtle awareness.'

'You are an Alexander Technique teacher!' exclaimed Dr Karen Gajda. 'Very pleased to meet you. I haven't had lessons but I read the book and taught it to myself. It helped me set my records.' This was in the early 1980s, and the slim, blonde woman greeting me was visiting a group of osteopathic physicians in Chicago where I had begun to teach the Technique as a conservative, supplementary approach for patients with back pain.

The idea that Dr Gajda had 'taught herself the Alexander Technique' rankled but her tone was friendly, easy-going and full of energy. I smiled, shook her hand and wondered: 'What book?' 'What records?' Later, I learned that she won the women's title at the 1980 World Powerlifting Federation Championships. She set world records for her weight classification of 60kg (132lb) in the squat (162.5kg/356lb) and in the deadlift (170kg/374.5lb).

Her first actual lesson was limited to only 15 minutes. To start, I put my hands on her upper back. She asked, 'Oh, do you want me to release the rhomboids [the muscles between the spine and shoulder blades]?' Before I could say anything, her shoulder blade perceptibly moved. She did not seem to be tensing, forcing or anticipating. When she moved a body part to a new position, she did not set herself stiffly. Indeed, her muscles were alive to the touch.

It turned out that the book Dr Gadja had read on the Alexander Technique was Frank Pierce Jones's *Body Awareness in Action*. Jones had made a number of physical and psychometric measures of students before and during Alexander Technique lessons, which included tracking the head trajectory and the amounts of force exerted through the feet during the movement from sitting to standing. Without Alexander training,

Jones observed, the students tended to over-tense their necks and retract their heads. The force patterns exerted through the feet suggested unnecessary effort.

Dr Gajda's interest in Jones's studies was that the stand-to-sit movement is essentially a squat – which, in turn, is basic to all physical activity, such as a plié in dance, the ready position in tennis, or preparation for a golf swing. It engages multiple muscle groups in the back, legs and arms. She and her trainer had constructed a training system and a theory for optimal squat form. When applied to the squat, electromyographic studies had shown that the back extensor support muscles reciprocally inhibit automatically when a person flexes their torso too far forward during a squat. This can put the soft tissue of the back at considerable risk, especially when lifting heavy weights. Thus, it is vital for a powerlifter to learn to flex the hips and legs without flexing the torso – that is, to lift with a straight back. This is essentially the form taught in Alexander lessons.

Conventional powerlifter squat form, however, usually also includes hyperextending the neck and head, what Alexander teachers would call 'pulling the head back and down'. In contrast, Dr Gajda and her trainer interpreted the Jones studies to show that head hyperextension during a squat is a counterproductive habit rather than a protective requirement. Hence, she trained consciously to inhibit any tendency toward head/neck hyperextension during a lift, to direct her head 'forward and up'. Learning not to pull her head back during the squat, she said, was her competitive edge and helped achieve more consistently coordinated movement.

What the Alexander Technique brings to resistance training is subtle awareness, an attention to detail that can both enliven the process and help to prevent the bad habits that lead to injury. The focus is not on the end of lifting more, but the means of getting there.

Ed Bouchard

'If I don't grip my neck and freeze up at the joint between my spine and skull, everything begins to flow.'

I am a dancer and choreographer. I have been studying the Alexander Technique for almost two decades and teaching it for five years at studios throughout New York, including the Energy Center in Brooklyn where I also practise yoga.

Perhaps yoga is so popular because, like me, people want to be engaged as a whole person when they are exercising. Yoga provides an alternative to 'rote' exercising, which doesn't require a person's presence. Yoga is equal parts mental and physical; it asks that for an hour or so you consciously focus on what you are doing. Where else do you get such a chance? The Alexander Technique supports this approach because it is essentially a mind-body process that makes 'concentration' an expansive experience instead of a narrowing one. The Alexander principles address the very real problem of how we do what we do; they assume that unity of the self is possible now, in this moment, whether you have the posture right or not. They give you a way to develop the stamina to be present, the stamina to have fun.

Having fun is very practical for me. Each time I do an asana, it can be a new experience as long as I use awareness, inhibition and direction. If I am willing to relinquish my idea of what I should do, and to imagine my movement happening in a new way, my practice is full of kinetic surprises. Sometimes I just have to laugh at how much easier a posture is than I thought it would be. Very specifically, if I don't grip my neck and freeze up at the joint between my spine and skull, everything begins to flow. I always give myself permission not to do a posture if I can't manage to free my neck somewhere in there. This very simple awareness helps me to define the edge between challenge and injury – I have never hurt myself in a yoga class since I began my Alexander training. I now know when to back off, and when to go for it.

Most people, me included, tend to compress their joints forcefully when they push, reach or make a shape. This is the cause of many injuries. Pulling is an essential transitional movement in getting from one posture to the next, and usually it needs to be very well coordinated with a push and a reach. If you can feel compression, then you can make a choice before initiating a movement to 'un-compress'. Hence, the other thing that I help my students with is to notice when they are compressing. That attention is a window of opportunity in which to choose another option. Instead of right and wrong, you can just do it differently.

Here is an example of what I mean. In the effort to achieve a shape, and especially when bearing weight on the arms, many people will tense or pull up their shoulders. The most common correction for that would be to 'pull the shoulders down' or 'pull the shoulders back towards each other and open your chest'. However, that's just adding an extra problem to the original problem: not only are you holding your shoulders up, but you're now trying to pull down against the holding up.

Instead of fighting yourself this way, all you really have to do is give up the original holding. Then wish for your whole arm to release away from your torso, towards the floor. If you can notice compressive movement habits, you won't have to use them as a response to movement challenges and you should avoid injuring yourself.

When you're not wasting energy fighting yourself, you can focus on the posture at hand and allow the energy to flow through you. Even one or two moments like that in a class can be wonderfully exhilarating.

Clare Maxwell

CONCLUSION: PAST, PRESENT – FUTURE?

'I bought all those Jane Fonda videos. I love to sit and eat cookies and watch 'em.'

Dolly Parton

It's incredible to think that 35 years ago, there was no such thing as a 'fitness industry' and Britain boasted a mere handful of sports centres. Only 25 years ago, the aerobics revolution had barely started. And little more than ten years ago, yoga and Pilates were still esoteric pursuits practised by the discerning few.

At the end of the 1970s, Dr Kenneth Cooper coined the term 'aerobics'. No, Jane Fonda didn't invent it; we battled through 'the burn' with her. We had the first great jogging boom, and a more recent re-evaluation of running as safe and effective physical activity for all ages. Then came the late 1980s fitness revolution, with clubs designed to meet the aspirations of the 'me generation', decked out in chrome and primary colours with a thumping sound system.

A reaction was inevitable, and the 1990s brought a new interest in 'holistic fitness'. The mechanical approach was replaced by a philosophy that placed mind, body and spirit as equal points on the exercise triangle. Suddenly, it seemed rather futile to spend half an hour pedalling on a bike with no wheels when fresh air and sunshine were but a short ride away. 'Natural' activities such as walking, rowing and outdoor swimming were promoted as an antidote to the potential tedium of an entirely indoor workout regime.

This change of emphasis also compelled fitness clubs to rethink their strategy. It was no longer acceptable to provide a weights room and an unvarying programme of high-intensity aerobics classes, and to demand a huge monthly direct debit for the privilege of membership. Increasing professionalism within the fitness industry, linked to higher expectations among customers, also played a part in powering this more enduring 'holistic' revolution in how we exercise.

The term 'holistic' comes from the Greek word for 'whole' and is used to describe any system, be it medicine or exercise, that considers the whole person – body, mind and spirit – within the wider environment of family, culture and community. The basic principles are that each individual is unique; that the psychosocial aspects of lifestyle and personal fulfilment are essential to good health; and that practitioner and client share equal responsibility for the success of the process. In the context of the gym, then, this means the role of the weights room supervisor is no longer about offering instruction to an exerciser in how to build big biceps, but about working together on a journey of psychophysical self-discovery.

Fascinating links have already been established between conventional fitness activities and a holistic approach, in *Master the Art of Swimming* by Steven Shaw and *Master the Art of Running* by Malcolm Balk and Andrew Shields. In both books, the authors ask whether swimming and running can be considered as arts rather than mere sports. They argue that they can, by downplaying the need to swim/run faster or further and instead learning to enjoy the process of the activity. For example, instead of making efficient swimming sound like rocket science and turning competitive swimming into a battle against an intransigent opponent, the pleasure of enhanced awareness in the water should be the reward of the activity. For Shaw, a competitive swimmer who quit the sport bored and exhausted, learning to check his competitive instincts and 'slow down' presented the challenge of discovering a new kind of self-control, what he describes as 'a sense of continuing exploration of the water and of myself'.

Likewise, for Malcolm Balk, 'Every run is different, and how I react to each run can be a matter of choice, or creation – staying present, responding intelligently to the situation, taking calculated risks, finding a different way to achieve my goal. When I tell runners that there is something new to be learned every time they put on their shoes, they sometimes look at me with disbelief. But the truth is that, even though I've been running for more than 25 years, I still feel like I learn something every day. It's not just a cliché, it's what feeds the process.'

The great athlete Filbert Bayi once said: 'From running I derive not just physical but aesthetic pleasure.' He meant that running can be considered an art and, with that in mind, it's worth pausing here to consider what the title of this book means.

Exercise is so often seen as a necessary evil, to be endured for the sake of health or a slimmer waistline. Such thinking can add exercise to the list of robotic, mundane activities that characterize so much of our lives. When we cut our minds off from what we are doing and simply repeat movements over and over, in a mechanical fashion, without interest or curiosity, without thought and without intention, we reduce both the experience and ourselves in the process. After all, who needs to spend more time at the office?!

The art of working out, then, is to be found in the process of exercising. And the beauty of this art is that it has to be recreated every time you set foot in the gym.

FURTHER READING AND SOURCES OF INFORMATION

Alexander Technique and its applications

Body Awareness in Action by Frank Pierce Jones (Schoken Books, 1979).

Body Learning by Michael Gelb (Aurum, 1994). An excellent introduction to the Alexander Technique.

Constructive Conscious Control of the Individual by F. Matthias Alexander (Gollancz, 1923).

Master the Art of Running by Malcolm Balk and Andrew Shields (Collins & Brown, 2006).

Master the Art of Swimming by Steven Shaw (Collins & Brown, 2006).

The Alexander Technique: A Skill for Life by Pedro de Alcantara (Crowood Press, 1999).

The Art of Changing by Glen Park (Ashgrove Publishing, 2000).

The Complete Illustrated Guide to the Alexander Technique by Glyn McDonald (Element, 1998).

The Use of the Self by F. Matthias Alexander (Gollancz, 1932).

The Alexander Principle by Wilfred Barlow (Gollancz, 1973).

Exercise, fitness and gym culture

Bench Press by Sven Lindqvist (Granta Books, 2003). A poetic meditation on gym culture and history.

Facts and Fallacies of Fitness by Mel Siff (Self-published, 1995). Healthy scepticism backed up by immense theoretical and practical knowledge.

'FlowMotion' series: *Pilates* by Suzanne Scott, *Stretching* by Simon Frost, *Tai Chi* by James Drewe, *Yoga* by Liz Lark (Connections Book Publishing, 2002). Digital wide-format photographs capture entire movement sequences.

Full Strength by Werner Kieser (Martin Dunitz, 2000). Authoritative strength training manual.

Fusion Fitness by Chan Ling Yap (A&C Black, 2002). Interesting ideas on blending Eastern and Western exercise disciplines.

The Health & Fitness Handbook by Julia Dalgleish and Stuart Dollery (Longman, 2001). Comprehensive text for exercise professionals.

The Owner's Guide to the Body by Roger Golten (Thorsons, 1999.) Increasing body awareness through the principles of Hellerwork.

The Stark Reality of Stretching by Dr Steven D. Stark (Independent Publishers Group, 1997). A well-written and user-friendly introduction.

YMCA Guide to Exercise to Music by Rodney Cullum and Lesley Mowbray (Pelham, 1986). The first book published on the subject and still a standard reference for students.

Health

Fat Land: How Americans Became the Fattest People in the World by Greg Critser (Penguin, 2003).

Handbook for the Urban Warrior by Barefoot Doctor (Thorsons, 2000).

The Art of Effortless Living by Ingrid Bacci (Bantam Books, 2000).

Ultimate Health by Dr John Briffa (Michael Joseph, 2002).

Pilates

Pilates Body Power by Lesley Ackland (Thorsons, 2001).

Ultimate Pilates by Dreas Reyneke (Vermilion, 2002).

Running

Once A Runner by John L Parker Jr. (Cedarwinds Publishing, 1978.) The greatest book ever written on running!

Pose Method of Running by Dr Nicholas Romanov with John Robson (Dr Romanov's Sport Education Series, 2002).

Run for Life: The Real Woman's Guide to Running by Sam Murphy (Kyle Cathie, 2003).

Yoga

Are You A Natural Hatha Yogi? by Ken Thompson (Angela's Yoga Books, 2002), available in the UK from 01603 872030.

The Easy Yoga Workbook by Tara Fraser (Duncan Baird Publishers, 2003). Includes a useful section on 'easy yoga for easy sports'.

Journey into Power by Baron Baptiste (Thorsons, 2002).

Power Yoga by Beryl Bender Birch (Prion Books, 1995). By the wellness director and yoga teacher in residence of the New York Road Runners' Club.

Websites

<www.artofswimming.com> Steven Shaw's Alexander Technique-inspired approach to swimming.

<www.chekinstitute.com> A great website with useful articles on many aspects of fitness.

<www.dryessis.com> Articles and products relating to many aspects of exercise, fitness, nutrition and training.

<www.posetech.com> An excellent site for anyone interested in running.

<www.rrnews.com> An informative monthly journal that goes well beyond running, with topics including cross-training, mental preparation, nutrition and stretching.

<www.theartofrunning.com> Information on the book *Master the Art of Running*, by Malcolm Balk and Andrew Shields, plus details of workshops in the UK, Canada, USA, Australia and Europe.

CONTRIBUTORS

David Bainbridge is an Alexander Technique teacher based in Wiltshire.
davbat@totalise.co.uk

Ed Bouchard has taught the Alexander Technique since 1979 and is a co-founder of AmSAT. He has a Masters degree in Public Health from the University of Illinois. He wrote *Kinesthetic Ventures* with his Alexander Technique student Ben Wright and teacher Michael Protzel.
ed@ATeducationresearch.com

Max Bower is a full-time freelance exercise instructor. He also works as an exercise instructor on University College London Hospital's Cardiac Rehabilitation scheme, and developed an exercise foundation course for cardiac rehabilitation nurses in conjunction with Dr Jenny Bell of the British Association for Cardiac Rehabilitation.
m.bower@ymcafit.org.uk

Alison Broome is an Alexander Technique teacher living in the Lake District. She applies the Technique to her work, hill-walking, cycling and now skills in parenthood!
alison.marsden@integratinghealth.com

Clare Canning is fitness training director at Central YMCA in London. She is responsible for developing training courses for personal trainers and fitness instructors in the concept and use of core stability exercises and equipment both in class and one-to-one settings.
c.canning@centralymca.org.uk

Myra David holds degrees in physical education and counselling. A lifetime student of dance and movement, she has trained with Les Grands Ballets Canadiens, Les Ballets Jazz and as an integrative yoga therapist. She has more than 30 years' teaching experience at Vanier College in Montreal.
davidm@vaniercollege.qc.ca

Erica Donnison graduated from the Fellside Alexander Technique Training School in Kendal, Cumbria, in July 2004. She is interested in applying the Technique to sports performance, particularly cycling and running.
ericad@zetnet.co.uk

Fred Horowitz is a business coach in Quebec, working with small business owners who are frustrated with the growth of their organization and the cost that their hard work has on the quality of their lives.
fhorow@videotron.ca

Carol Levin is a published poet and literary manager of the Art Theatre of Puget Sound. She is a member of the Executive Board of Alexander Technique International and studies the Technique in Seattle, Washington.
clevin@televar.com

Clare Maxwell received her certification as a teacher from the American Center for Alexander Technique (ACAT) in New York City, where she has a lively private practice. She is a member of the volunteer faculty at ACAT and teaches Alexander Technique and movement workshops nationally. Clare brings to her practice more than 20 years of experience as a dancer and choreographer.
claremax@mindspring.com or
www.claremaxwell.com

Denise McKeever is an Alexander Technique teacher based near Detroit. She is also certified in Pilates and Gyrotonic.
denisemckeever@comcast.net

Patrick Pearson teaches the Alexander Technique in the Welsh Marches and coaches rowing at Pengwern Boat Club in Shrewsbury and elsewhere in the UK. He specializes in applying the Alexander Technique to rowing and has worked with all levels of athlete from club competitors to Olympians. He also runs workshops for rowers, coaches, Alexander Technique teachers and students.
patrickalexrow@hotmail.com

Robin Simmons is based in Zurich, where he runs an Alexander Technique training school and gives lessons. He has studied tai chi since 1969.
simmons.heiz@bluewin.ch

Madelene Webb is an Alexander Technique teacher in central and north London. She has been involved in university trials being conducted into the role of the Technique, exercise and massage in alleviating back pain.
madelene@nopain-gain.com

Brigitte Wrenn is exercise to music director at Central YMCA in London. She has developed the YMCA Cardiokick and YMCA Supple Strength courses and is also a tutor for YMCA Fitness Industry Training.
b.wrenn@centralymca.org.uk

PICTURE CREDITS

Page 19 © EMPICS
Page 20 © Getty Images Sport
Page 33 © PHOTOGRAPH BY TOM BLAU, CAMERA PRESS LONDON
Page 49 © EMPICS
Page 51 © Ken Kaminesky/Take 2 Productions/Corbis
Page 53 © EMPICS
Page 69 © Brand X Pictures/Alamy
Page 81 © EMPICS
Page 102-103 © Patrick Pearson
Page 109 © EMPICS
Page 111 © Ruediger Knobloch/A.B./zefa/Corbis
Page 117 © LWA-JDC/CORBIS
Page 128 © Getty Images Sport
Page 140 © EMPICS
Page 141© EMPICS

INDEX